IMMUNISATION IN PRACTICE

IMMUNISATION IN PRACTICE

S.K.MITTAL
Associate Professor
Department of Pediatrics
Maulana Azad Medical College, New Delhi

S.KUKREJA
Consultant Pediatrician
Batra Hospital & Medical Research Centre
New Delhi

CBS

CBS Publishers & Distributors Pvt. Ltd.

New Delhi • Bengaluru • Chennai • Kochi • Kolkata • Mumbai
Hyderabad • Nagpur • Patna • Pune • Vijayawada

Second Edition: 1996
Reprint: 1998, 1999, 2000, 2001, 2002,
2003, 2004, 2006, 2010, 2016

Published by:
Satish Kumar Jain for CBS Publishers & Distributors Pvt. Ltd.,
4819/XI Prahlad Street, 24 Ansari Road, Daryaganj, New Delhi - 110002
delhi@cbspd.com, cbspubs@airtelmail.in • www.cbspd.com
Ph.: 23289259, 23266861, 23266867 • Fax: 011-23243014

Corporate Office: 204 FIE, Industrial Area, Patparganj, Delhi - 110 092
Ph: 49344934 • Fax: 011-49344935
E-mail: publishing@cbspd.com • publicity@cbspd.com

Branches:
- ***Bengaluru:*** 2975, 17th Cross, K.R. Road, Bansankari 2nd Stage, Bengaluru - 70 • Ph: +91-80-26771678/79 • Fax: +91-80-26771680 E-mail: cbsbng@gmail.com, bangalore@cbspd.com
- ***Chennai:*** No. 7, Subbaraya Street, Shenoy Nagar, Chennai - 600030 Ph: +91-44-26681266, 26680620 • Fax: +91-44-42032115 E-mail: chennai@cbspd.com
- ***Kochi:*** Ashana House, 39/1904, A.M. Thomas Road, Valanjambalam. Ernakulum, Kochi • Ph: +91-484-4059061-65 Fax: +91-484-4059065 • E-mail: cochin@cbspd.com
- ***Kolkata:*** 6-B, Ground Floor, Rameshwar Shaw Road, Kolkata - 700014 Ph: +91-33-22891126/7/8 • E-mail: kolkata@cbspd.com
- ***Mumbai:*** 83-C, Dr. E. Moses Road, Worli, Mumbai - 400018 Ph: +91-9833017933, 022-24902340/41 • E-mail: mumbai@cbspd.com

Representatives:
- Hyderabad: 0-9885175004
- Patna: 0-9334159340
- Vijayawada: 0-9000660880
- Nagpur: 0-9021734563
- Pune: 0-9623451994

Printed at:
J.S. Offset Printers, Delhi

PREFACE

There is a lot of confusion in translating principles of immunization into clinical practice. Epidemiological compulsions and economic constraints have compelled the W.H.O. and Government of India to suggest immunization schedules which are not in conformity with those practised in the developed countries. Doctors are often confronted with demanding parents who would have nothing but the best for their children. Confusion is further aggravated because different institutions and pediatricians follow different schedules in their practice. In absence of a thorough understanding of the efficacy and limitations of each immunising agent, a large number of questions remain unanswered in the minds of medical personnel. In trying to synthesise the variously practised schedules in his clinical practice, he is often compelled to follow his own schedule which may not even be optimal. Clear cut guide-lines on storage, transport of vaccines and special situations in which various vaccines and immunoglobulins may be used are not easily available in commonly available text books. This volume has been specially compiled to serve as a ready reference to the medical personnel for their day to day problems regarding immunisations arising in their clinical practice.

Opinions of different experts have been synthesised in this volume and where ever required, fully explained, so that the reader can understand the reasons behind these opinions. Where considered necessary, editorial comments (in italics) have been added to further clarify the differing opinions.

The book at places may appear repetitious but this is unavoidable as different practitioners see the same problem from different angles.

We hope that the reader would find this a useful ready reference book for their day to day problems.

New Delhi
Dated : 23rd Jan. 1991

S. K. Mittal
S. Kukreja

CONTRIBUTORS

Dr. Agarwal, Vijay
Consultant Pediatrician
Member, Immunization Advisory Committee
Indian Academy of Pediatrics
New Delhi.

Dr. Arya, Subhash
Consultant Pediatrician
Sir Ganga Ram Hospital
New Delhi.

Dr. Desai, A.B.
Chairman, Immunization Advisory Committee
Indian Academy of Pediatrics
Ahmedabad.

Dr. Dutta, A.K.
Assoc. Professor of Pediatrics
Member, Immunization Advisory Committee
Indian Academy of Pediatrics
Kalawati Saran Children's Hospital
New Delhi.

Dr. John, Jacob
Prof. & Head, Deptt. of Virology
Christian Medical College & Hospital
Vellore.

Dr. Kumar, Lata
Additional Prof. of Pediatrics
P.G.I., Chandigarh.

Dr. Kukreja, Shyam
Consultant Pediatrician
Batra Hospital,
New Delhi.

Dr. Meharban Singh
Prof. & Head, Deptt. of Pediatrics
A.I.I.M.S.
New Delhi.

Dr. Mittal, S.K.
Assoc. Prof. of Pediatrics
Member, Immunization Advisory Committee
Indian Academy of Pediatrics
M.A.M.C., LNJPN Hospital,
New Delhi.

Dr. Parthasarathy, A
Assoc. Prof. of Pediatrics
Madras Medical College,
Member, Immunization Advisory Committee
Indian Academy of Pediatrics
Madras.

Dr. Puri, R.K.
Prof. & Head,
Deptt. of Pediatrics,
M.A. Medical College & LNJPN Hospital
New Delhi.

Dr. Seth, Vimlesh
Professor of Pediatrics
A.I.I.M.S.,
New Delhi.

Dr. Shah, Raju C.
Consultant Pediatrician
Member, Immunization Advisory Committee
Indian Academy of Pediatrics
Ahmedabad.

Dr. Sharma, Daya
Professor of Pediatrics
Kalawati Saran Children's Hospital
New Delhi.

Dr. Taneja, Arvind
Consultant Pediatrician
Batra Hospital,
New Delhi.

CONTENTS

IMMUNISATION: GENERAL CONSIDERATIONS

Dr. S. Kukreja & Dr. S.K. Mittal

Q.1. How important is the role of immunization in control of infectious diseases ?

Immunization plays a very important role in control of infectious diseases. They help to build up immunity in the immunized individuals against specific diseases and thus help to decrease the transmission of diseases from one person to another. Successful eradication of small-pox is a shining example of how immunization can be used to eradicate an infectious disease.

However it must be remembered that the incidence of most of the infectious diseases in the developed countries was largely controlled even before many of the vaccines became available (Fig. 1). This was achieved by implementing simple public health measures like

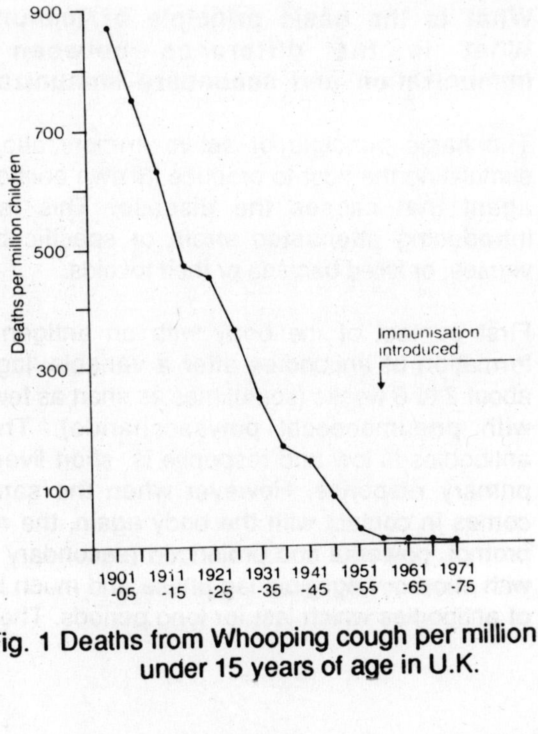

Fig. 1 Deaths from Whooping cough per million children under 15 years of age in U.K.

sanitation, water supply, proper housing etc. As the role of asepsis in surgery continues to be important despite availability of potent antibiotics, so does the role of public health measures continue to be important in this era of immunization.

Q.2. What is the meaning of vaccine and vaccination? What is the difference between vaccination and immunisation ?

Originally the vaccine word was used for cow pustule material which was used by Jenner to render humans immune to small pox. Consequently the method was called vaccination. Over the years, the meaning of these two words has broadened. Now vaccine means any immunological product used in active immunisation of humans and animals and the words vaccination & immunisation are used interchangeably. Immunisation can be active or passive,while vaccination is always active.

Q.3. What is the basic principle of immunization ? What is the difference between primary immunization and secondary immunization ?

The basic principle of active immunization involves stimulating the host to produce its own antibodies to the agent that causes the disease. This is done by introducing attenuated strain of specific bacteria or viruses, or killed bacteria or their toxoids.

First contact of the body with an antigen results in formation of antibodies after a variable 'lag phase' of about 2 to 6 weeks (sometimes as short as few hours like with pneumococcal polysaccharide). The titre of antibodies is low and response is short lived. This is a primary response. However when the same antigen comes in contact with the body again, the response is prompt, powerful and prolonged (secondary response), with short or negligible lag phase and much higher level of antibodies which last for long periods. The antibodies formed in the primary response are predominantly IgM and in secondary response, IgG. (Fig 2.)

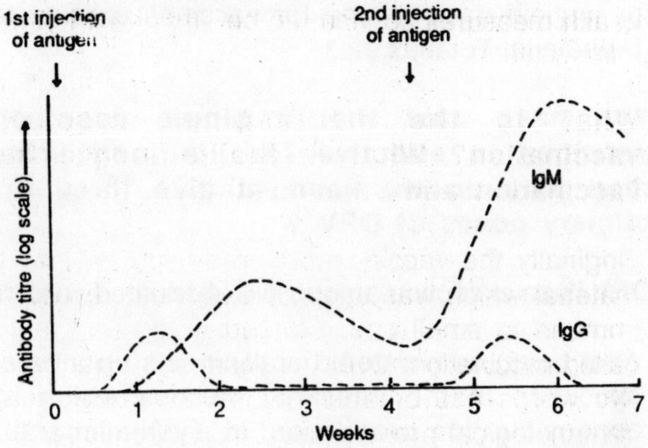

Fig. 2 Synthesis of IgG and IgM antibodies in Primary and secondary immune responses to antigens

Q.4. Why is it that for live vaccine (BCG, measles), we use only one dose of primary immunisation, while we give 2 or 3 primary doses of killed vaccine (Typhoid, DPT) vaccine ? Why are the 2nd and 3rd primary doses not called as boosters ?

Whenever a live vaccine (BCG and measles) is administered, the live attenuated (vaccine) organisms set up an infection (similar to natural infection) in the recipient and replicate, leading to ongoing antigenic stimulation which acts as both primary and secondary immunization and prolongs the antibody response. Also, this ensures that almost all recipients are effectively seroconverted with even one dose of live vaccine, given in most ideal circumstances (age of the host & vaccine potency etc) or adequately primed for any further immunological challenge.

In case of killed vaccines, to ensure adequate seroconversion in all individuals, a very large amount of antigen is required as this does not replicate on its own, (e.g 60-80 million killed bacilli are required for effective immunization against pertussis). This can not be given in a single dose because of markedly increased side effects. Therefore the dose is divided into three doses to achieve adequate seroconversion. Same holds true for typhoid vaccine and for vaccines utilising toxoids (Diphtheria, Tetanus etc.)

Q.5. You have said that a single dose of live vaccines is effective for life long immunity, then why do we need to give three or four primary doses of OPV ?

OPV is an exception among live attenuated vaccines.

After being administered orally it sets up a process of replication in the intestinal mucosa which is then responsible for production of systemic antibodies against it. Because of adverse circumstances in the gut (other entero viruses replicating) this vaccine virus may not always be able to replicate and that particular dose may not have any effect (acting like a 'hit' or miss' vaccine). Further, OPV is a trivalent vaccine containing three serotypes of polio virus. Usually only one of the serotypes is able to get a foothold in the intestine and does not allow other two serotypes to achieve replication at the same time. Thus, to ensure seroconversion against all the three serotypes, in maximum number of recipients, multiple doses of trivalent OPV are required.

Q.6. Why do some authorities recommend giving a second dose of measles vaccine despite the fact that this is a live attenuated viral vaccine ?

If the measles vaccine is given after 15 months of age then there is no interference to the replication of measles vaccine virus by maternal antibodies and a second dose is not required. But when the vaccine is given earlier than one year of age (more so before 9 months), persistance of maternal antibodies does not allow replication of measles vaccine virus. In such cases second dose of measles is required after 15 months of age (For details see Chapter on Measles & MMR).

Q.7. What is the most ideal (immunological) interval between three doses of DPT vaccine. Do we practice it? If not, Why ?

From the immunological point of view, the most ideal interval between 1st & 2nd dose of DPT is 2 months while between the 2nd and 3rd dose is 6 months. Because of the compelling need of completing the schedule as early as possible (especially against pertussis) and to improve compliance, this schedule can not be followed in practice. The recommended interval of 4 to 8 weeks is a satisfactory compromise between the biological basis of immune response and the need of completing the schedule as early as possible.

Q.8. Whenever there is lapse of even more than 6 months after the Ist dose of DPT, restarting of schedule in not recommended, why so ?

Whenever an antigen is injected in the body a clone of lymphocytes against the particular antigen is formed in the body. These converted lymphocytes produce antibodies and act as effector cells (Fig. 3.). In addition, a small number of memory cells are also produced in the

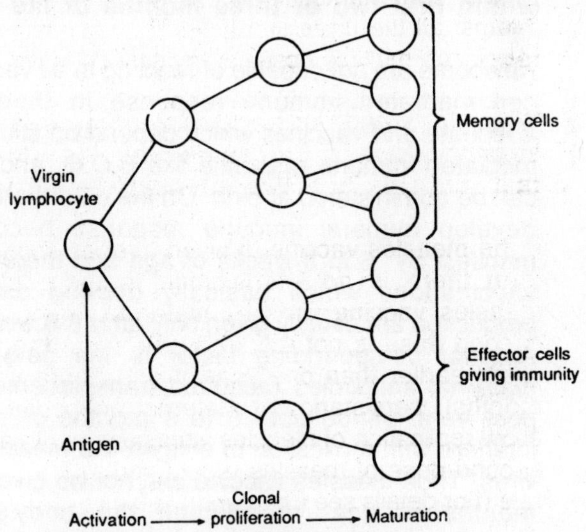

Fig. 3 Cellular basis of primary immune response

body. Whenever the antigen is reintroduced in the body, these 'memory cells' are able to produce effector cells and through them the specific antibodies. This immunological memory once introduced is almost never lost. It is because of this reason that irrespective of the lapse of time after the previous dose, the schedule is never required to be restarted again.

Q.9. Why are vaccinations recommended mostly in early childhood ?

Children not having been exposed to different infections, are highly susceptible to develop these infections. The aim of immunization is to prevent the persons from getting the disease when they are exposed to it for the first time in life as the first exposure itself may be crippling or fatal. Hence most of the vaccinations are given in early infancy.

Early vaccination also helps to prevent spread of infection in the community as it brings down the number of susceptible individuals in the community.

Q.10. Why we do not give all the vaccines at birth or within first two or three months of life ?

Newborns are not capable of reacting to all vaccines. The cell mediated immune response in them is quite adequate and vaccines which depend on stimulated cell mediated immune response like B.C.G. and small pox can be administered at birth. On the other hand, ability to develop humoral immune response becomes fully manifest by 6 to 8 weeks of age and therefore, those vaccinations which basically depend on antibody production are usually given only after 6-8 weeks of age. Another compounding factor is the persistence of maternal antibodies (acquired transplacentally) in the post natal period upto 6 to 9 months of age, which interfere with replication of antigen like measles vaccine virus. Thus measles vaccine can not be given before 6 months of age. In addition the body's immune mechanism is incapable of recognizing certain antigens (polysaccharide antigens of *pneumococcus, meningococcus & H. influenzae*) before two years of age and hence these vaccines can not be given before that age.

Q.11. How is the efficacy of a vaccine assessed ?

The most important parameter of vaccine efficacy is its capability to prevent natural infection in the recipient. During the development of a vaccine it is usually first ensured that the vaccine is effective in susceptible species of animals and then it is approved for human studies. The later require large field trials involving double blind controls for assessing the efficacy, (by comparing the rate of illness in unimmunised and immunized population) and safety in the human being. It is only after satisfactory human trials, that the vaccine is released for general use.

However in routine practice, it is not possible to judge the efficacy of the vaccine by demonstrating such clinical effectiveness. For this purpose, immunological effectiveness i.e the capacity of the vaccine to produce protective levels of antibodies, is generally utilised as an index of vaccine efficacy in short term trials. This however may not always correlate with clinical efficacy. Thus while immunological response may be demonstrable after some vaccines, (notably Typhoid) yet the protection provided in face of a large infectious dose may not be adequate. On the other hand, the clinical efficacy provided by say, one dose of measles may be greater than that suggested by the seroconversion, as the immunological system gets primed, (without adequate antibody response) and responds adequately to any future infectious challenge.

Q.12. What is the most effective route of administration of a vaccine ?

In general the most effective route of administration of any vaccine is the route followed by the natural infection as it largely simulates the host response in exactly the same manner as seen in natural infection. It has been shown that protection against common respiratory pathogens e.g., Influenza virus, correlate better with the presence of IgA associated antibodies in the respiratory passages than with the circulating IgG antibodies. Similarly O.P.V. is generally superior to I.P.V. as it provides local gut immunity (and also "herd immunity", which the killed vaccine is not able to do.

However, the natural route of infection is not always easy to follow for vaccine administration. Thus inhaled vaccines are generally very difficult to administer in actual clinical practice esp. to young infants and hence we have to depend on comparatively less effective but practical routes (I.M. or S.C.) of administration.

Comparative studies have also revealed that for some vaccines, (D.P.T., Typhoid), intradermal route may be more efficacious requiring 1/3rd to 1/10th of the dose required in the subcutaneos route. But the intradernal route has not found acceptance (except for BCG) because of limited data and because of intense local reaction which it may produce.

Q.13. Why do we insist on mass coverage of the community with different vaccines ? Many parents do not want their children to be vaccinated. Why should we insist that they get the vaccinations?

Vaccines prevent the diseases only in vaccinated children, so the parents must be told that this is for their child's own good that they should have him vaccinated. Mass vaccination campaign has the advantage for the whole community because by ensuring large number of immune individuals, we help to decrease the number of susceptible individuals in the community (Herd effect), because of which infecting bacteria or viruses are not able to get transmitted to another susceptible host. Thus community coverage not only ensures individual protection but also controls & eradicates the infection.

One of the most important effects of simultaneous mass vaccination of OPV (pulse immunization) is that it helps to curb the circulation of wild polio virus in the community by replacing it with the vaccine virus. This has been found to be the most effective way of eradicating polio from the community in shortest possible time.

Q.14. What are the advantages and disadvantages of live and killed vaccine ?

Live attenuated vaccines are extremely potent and usually produce life long immunity even with one injection (measles, mumps, rubella). They however have the disadvantage that they can not be given to immunocompromised individuals, whether because of disease (Hypogamma globullmenia,Lukemia, Lymphoma etc) or drugs (Corticosteroids, immuno-suppressants etc.,). There is also a potential danger of transmitting vaccine virus to a susceptible immunocompromised contact of the vaccine and thus cause vaccine virus induced disease in the contact (e.g.OPV). A live attenuated vaccine has a theoretical risk of possible activation in the host and there by causing the disease as happened earlier with BCG vaccine. The other disadvantage is that these vaccines need stringent storage & transport conditions.

Killed vaccines do not suffer from these disadvantages and they are by and large safe. However they make comparatively poor immunogenic agents, usually requiring multiple doses for adequate protection. These vaccines are only capable of providing individual protection and do not help to produce the 'herd effect' (IPV vs OPV).

Q.15. Why few "established" vaccines are no longer recommended or used e.g. small pox, cholera, & nerve tissue vaccine against rabies.

Small Pox is no more recommended because the disease has been completely eradicated. Today the risk due to small pox vaccination is much higher than that due to contracting the disease.

Cholera vaccine is ineffective as proved by several studies. If cholera is introduced into UK or USA, it is unlikely to spread because of high standards of public health practices. Even if highly effective cholera vaccine was available there, there will be no question of using it in mass campaigns. In any case the available cholera vaccine is a very poor vaccine and hence this is no more recommended.

Never tissue vaccine (NTV) against rabies has serious side effects. Serious reactions could be acceptable with a vaccine designed to prevent a disease with high morbidity and mortality. As rabies is uniformly fatal, nerve tissue vaccine was acceptable in cases of post exposure prophylaxis. With the advent of newer vacccines (HDCV,PCEC) which are much safer and highly effective, the NTV is no more recommended. (See chapter on Rabies).

Q.16. Can we administer two or three vaccines simultaneously ? It is said that two live virus vaccines should not be given concurrently. Kindly highlight this aspect.

Certain vaccines are frequently given at the same time in childhood especially in those children who report late for vaccination. Simultaneous administration of vaccine saves visits and hence helps greatly in improving vaccine coverage. Serological surveys and field observations indicate that simultaneous administration of most of the vaccines has not resulted in impaired antibody response or increased rates of adverse reactions.

Different live vaccines can also be administered simultaneously but not at different times within one month because the active replication of first vaccine virus might interfere with uptake and replication of the second. Therefore, a gap of at least one month should be kept between two vaccinations, if they cannot be given at the same time.

Q.17. What is the role of vaccines in epidemics ?

In case of a threat of epidemic, emergency mass immunisation may be carried out to rapidly build up immunity and to interrupt the transmission of the disease. For example, in case of a polio epidemic, mass immunization will lead to replication of polio virus strain in the guts of the recipients and thus will prevent transmission of the wild virus. Other vaccines which can be used to control epidemics are meningococcal, measles, yellow fever and influenza vaccine. Cholera vaccine has no role in epidemic situations.

Q.18. Can a malnourished child be given vaccination?

Yes it has been established by many studies that the capacity of malnourished children to establish a humoral immune response is largely intact and they can be successfully immunized with vaccines like DPT, typhoid, measles, OPV etc.

Even BCG is a capable of evoking a CMI response in malnourished children and hence can be given safely to them.

Bibliography

1. Adams JM The organisation and experession of immunoglobulin genes immunology today, 1980, 1:10.
2. Avrameas S, Antonie JC, Ternynk T. Development of immunoglobulin and antibody forming cells in different stages of the immune response. Ann. Immunol. 1976, 127,551.
3. AJJan N. Vaccination. Institute Merieux France.
4. Cooke JV et al . Antibody formation in early infancy against diptheria and tetanus toxids. J Ped 1948. 133:

5. Centers for disease Control. General recommendations on immunization. MMWR 1983, 32.1.
6. Chandra RK. Interaction of nutrition, infection and immune response: immunocompetence in nutritional deficiency, methodological considerations and intervention strategies. Acta Paediatr. Scand. 1977, 68, 137.
7. Dick G. Immunisation Update. Books Publication UK 19788 Edition.
8. Ifekwunigwe AE Grasset N, Glass R, Roster S. Immune response to measles and smallpox vaccination in malnourished children. Amer. J. Clin. Nutr. 1980, 33: 621.
9. Mcgregor IA. Nutrition and immunization. Seminar on Immunization in Africa C.I.E. Fondation Merieux ed.; Kampala 1971, 198.
10. OMS-WHO. Immunological recognition and effector mechanism in infectious diseases (A WHO meeting). Bull, WHO, 1980, 58, 671.
11. WHO : Intervals between successive doses of killed vaccines: the persistence of immunological Wly epidem Rev 54: 388, 1979.
12. Wilkins J et ak agglutinin response to pertussis vaccine, Effect of dosage and interval. J. Ped 1971. 79.

IMMUNISATION SCHEDULES 2

Dr. S.K. Mittal & Dr. S. Kukreja

Q.1. Why is the immunization schedule changed so often ? Is it really necessary ?

Immunization schedule of any country or community depends on the disease epidemiology, availability of vaccine, economic constraints, logistic problems and advent of newer vaccines. As many of these factors differ from country to country and from time to time in the same country, the immunisation schedule needs to be revised periodically. This is best examplified by the immunisation schedules followed by USA in 1964 (Table I) and in 1989 (Table II).

Table 1. Recommended Immunization Schedule—1964*

AGE	TYPE OF VACCINE
2 months	DPT, OPV 1
3 months	DPT, OPV 3
4 months	DPT, OPV 2
7 months	Smallpox
9 months	Measles vaccine (and human gamma globulin)
15 months	DPT, TVOPV
4 years	DPT
6 years	Smallpox
8 years	Td
11 years	Smallpox
12 years	Td
16 years	Td
Every 5 years after initial vaccination	T, smallpox

* Adapted from Nelson WE : textbook of Pediatrics, ed 8. Philadelphia, WB Saunders, 1964, p 155.

In our country small pox having been eradicated, the vaccine was dropped from the schedule (changing epidemiology). The age for vaccination with DPT was shifted to 6 weeks because of logistic reasons (to correspond with the post natal visit of mother). Typhoid & cholera vaccines were dropped because it was considered that they are not very effective vaccines. Measles vaccine is being given at 9 months as a compromise between the need to prevent the disease in early infancy and the need for effective seroconversion with a single dose. MMR is not being introduced in the country because of economic reasons.

Thus, one would see that immunization schedule is not a static process but a dynamic one which is adapted to suit the current needs of a community or a country.

Q.2. Many of the factors you mention, as determinants of immunization schedule in a country, are similar in most of the developed countries. Why is it that the immunization schedule is different in U.K. and U.S.A. also ?

You are right that the immunization schedule being followed in U.K., & U.S.A. are different but essentially they are similar in nature. (Table II) Differences are essentially due to minor epidemiological differences. U.K. still needs to give BCG vaccine at 11-14 years because it still has a substantial incidence of tuberculosis (among immigrant Asian population). USA has adopted a policy of universal immunisation of all children with MMR. The rationale was that such a strategy would reduce the circulation of virus in the community, which posed a major risk to the pragnant women. In contrast, selective vaccination of prepubescent girls was the sole approach followed in UK due to cost effective reasons. However, recently UK has planned to introduce additional MMR at 15 months in their schedule & USA has introduced a booster of MMR at 11-14 years. (or at 4-6 years).

Table II
Immunization Schedule in U.S.A. and U.K.

U.S.A.		U.K.	
Age	*Vaccine*	*Age*	*Vaccine*
2 months	DPT + OPV	3 months	DPT + OPV
4 months	DPT + OPV	5 months	DPT + OPV
6 months	DPT + OPV	11 months	DPT + OPV
15 months	MMR	1-2 yrs	Measles
18 months	DPT + OPV+Hib	3-5 yrs	DT + OPV
4-6 yrs	DPT + OPV	10-13 YRS	BCG to Mx (-ve)
14-16 yrs	Td	11-14 yrs	Rubella (Girls)
		15-19 yrs	OPV/IPV + TT

Q.3. What is EPI & UIP? Why this change in nomenclature and what is the essential difference?

Expanded programme of immunisation (EPI) was launched by W.H.O. and subsequently by Government of India in 1978, to enhance immunisation coverage of children and pregnant mothers. Prior to this, although vaccinations were practised in the country, there was no system of evaluation and monitoring and no attempt at mass coverage at national level. With the introduction of EPI, for the first time a national effort was launched to immunize children and thus to control the communicable diseases. Under this programme efforts were also made to step up the manufacture and availability of different vaccines in the country and to strengthen the system of cold chain.

Universal programme of Immunization (UIP) was launched in 1985 with a view to further improve the vaccine coverage. It was mainly evolved to concentrate at children under one year of age and to ensure that all infants are protected against 6 diseases before they reach the age of 1 year. Definite targets were laid down and it was decided that by the year 1990, more than 85%

of infants will be vaccinated against these diseases. The programme is intensely monitored and is largely achieving its objectives. Under this programme, the country is also rapidly achieving self sufficiency in vaccine production.

Q.4. What is the currently recommended immunization schedule in the country ? Is it the same as recommended by W.H.O. and if not,why so ?

The recommended schedule of immunization by the Govt. of India under the UIP is shown in Table III. This is generally in line with that suggested by WHO under EPI. WHO has recently recommended that in addition to this schedule, children in developing countries (like India) should also get two more doses of OPV, one at birth and one at 9 months (with measles). This recommendation has been made only in the year 1987 and the Government of India is actively considering the feasibility of incorporating this in the national schedule.

Table III

Immunization Schedules, UIP India and Recommended by WHO Global Advisory Committee (EPI) 1987

	UIP (India)	WHO
Birth	BCG + OPV*	BCG + OPV
6 weeks	DPT + OPV	DPT + OPV
10 weeks	DPT + OPV	DPT + OPV
14 weeks	DPT + OPV	DPT + OPV
9 month	Measles	Measles + OPV**
18 months	DPT + OPV	DPT + OPV

* Neonatal OPV recommended for use in Metropolitan cities March, 1990.

** 5th Dose of OPV is suggested only where sero-conversion with 4 doses are poor.

Q.5. What do you think about the national schedule ? Is it not too much of a compromise?

The Immunization Advisory Committee of Indian Academy of Pediatrics has carefully evaluated the national schedule and has unanimously concluded that UIP has by and large failed to achieve its objectives. This is largely because of rather ineffective way in which various vaccines are being used in UIP. The major recommendations of the committee are mentioned in Table IV

Table IV
Immunization Schedule

(Recommended by Immunisation Advisory Committee IAP (1989)

Age	Vaccine
Birth	BCG + OPV
6-8 weeks (2m)	DPT + OPV/IPV
12-16 weeks (4m)	DPT + OPV/IPV
18-24 weeks (6m)	DPT + OPV/IPV
7-9 months (8m)	Measles
1 1/2-2 yrs (18m)	DPT + OPV, MMR
2 yrs +	Typhoid two doses at 1 month interval
4-5 yrs	DPT + OPV
5 yrs	BCG (to Mx -individuals)*

NB. Pulse immunization with two doses of OPV given one month apart, to all children under 5 years in addition to the routine OPV immunization.
*Optional

The committee found that the seroconversion rates with OPV are poor when 4 weeks interval is used. This is because the polio vaccine virus continues to replicate in the intestinal mucosa for upto 8 weeks during which time it does not allow the uptake of the 2nd dose. Earlier, people have recommended using 5 doses of OPV to improve seroconversion rates. The committee discovered that even studies from India and other tropical countries, have also shown as good seroconversion rates with 3 doses of OPV given at eight weeks intervals, as those achieved with five doses of OPV given at four weeks intervals. Also, this 8 weeks interval would be much better for DPT immunisation. Similar schedule of 2,4 & 6 months is being followed in the U.S.A & U.K.

The committee was overwhelmingly of the view that polio is unlikely to be eradicated by just stepping up OPV coverage even if the dose interval is enhanced. It recommended exploring the use of IPV in place of OPV. Three doses of IPV given at 2, 4 & 6 months would give life long immunity to the individual, thus obviating the need of any further doses. Also, it would avoid the problems of cold chain maintenance which seems to be almost insurmountable. The committee also suggested introduction of pulse immunisation with OPV, till such time that the IPV can be introduced in the national immunization schedule. This pulse immunization is to be practised in addition to 3 doses of OPV at 8 weeks interval, (For details of pulse immunization, see Chapter on Polio).

The committee was of the view that the practice of giving one dose of measles vaccine at nine months of age, allows a large number of cases of measles to occur in the community both before and after the measles injection. It therefore recommended that first dose of measles vaccine be given between 7-9 months of age, followed by another dose at 15-18 months. The second dose can be combined with mumps and rubella (MMR) which will ensure life long immunity against all 3 diseases. Committee noted with concern that at present there is no national programme of control of mumps, which though a milder disease, yet has a very high incidence and causes lots of morbidity and may be responsible for more than 10 million school days lost every year in the country.

The committee also looked into the neccessity of second booster of DPT at 4-5 yrs, which has been omitted from the national schedule since 1983. epidemiological evidence available with the committee suggested that pertussis is fairly prevalent in 5-9 year olds and this incidence is likely to increase if the 2nd booster is not given at 4 to 5 years. These children are a great source of infection in the community and to the younger siblings at home. Hence for the control of the disease it is essential that the 2nd booster of DPT be continued at 4-5 years.

Finally the committee also found the neccessity of restoring typhoid vaccine in the national schedule and suggested trials with AKD type of typhoid vaccine. As a significant number of cases of typhoid occur below 5 years of age, it is suggested to start vaccination with typhoid vaccine at 2 years of age with boosters every 3 years.

Most important aspect of IAP schedule is that it ensure 2 monthly visits of the child which can then be utilised for comprehensive child health care.

Q.6. What schedule should be followed for unimmunised children presenting for the first time after 1 year of age ?

The schedule for 1-5 year old, and more than 5 year old unimmunised children is mentioned in Table V.

Table V

Immunisation Schedule for Unimmunised Children

	1-5 yrs	*>5 yrs*
1st vist	BCG, DPT, OPV	DT,* Mx.
2nd vist (4-8 wk)	DPT , OPV	DT, BCG (if Mx-ve)
3rd vist (4-8 wk)	DPT, OPV, Measles	
1 yr later	DPT, OPV	DT
2-3 years	Typhoid 2 doses 4 wks intervals	Typhoid 2 doses at 4 wks interval

* Td if more than 10 years.

Q.7. Which common misconceptions lead to non completion of immunisation schedule ?

Large number of misconception still prevail not only among the general population but even among health professionals, which often lead to non completion of schedule. These are:

a) Mild cold/cough/diarrhea.
b) Prematurity.
c) concurrent antimicrobial therapy.
d) Breast feeding.
e) Nonspecific allergies.
f) Family history of seizures.
g) SIDS in the family.
h) Family history of adverse reactions to vaccine
i) Static neurological disease.

None of these conditions warrant postponment of immunisation but are frequently made excuse for the same.

BCG VACCINE

1. Contents: Freeze dried live attenuated Calmette Guerin strain of bovine *Mycobacterium tuberculosis*, 0.1 to 0.4 million viable bacilli per dose.
2. **Ideal age for initiating primary immunization:** At birth or at earliest contact.
3. **Schedule of primary vaccination :** Single dose.
4. **Booster** : Not recommended routinely. May be given to Mantoux negative (> 5 years).
5. **Dose** : 0.1 ml.
6. **Route of administration** : Intradermal
7. **Site of administration** : Left upper arm at deltoid insertion.
8. **Preparation of site of vaccination:** None required (DO NOT USE antiseptics)
9. **Instructions to the mother after vaccination:**
   - i) Raised wheal will disappear in 1 hour or so.
   - ii) No reaction like fever, malaise.
   - iii) Local reaction after 3-6 weeks with a nodule formation which ulcerates and heals by scarring.
10. **Protective efficacy** : Tuberculin conversion in almost 100%, clinical efficacy variable 0-80% in different studies.
11. **Contraindications** : None (possibly avoid after measles infection or vaccination and in immunocompromised individuals).
12. **Side effects** : Non healing ulcer and regional suppurative lymphadenitis.
13. **Complication** : Risk of tuberculous disease in immuno-compromised host.
14. **Storage** :
    - a) **Vaccine not in use**: +2 ° to +8° C in the middle compartment of refrigerator.
    - b) **During immunization** : i) Keep away from light ii) Use within 3 hours.
    - c) **In case of electricity failure** : Can be left in the fridge. It is viable for 1 month even at 37° C.

B C G VACCINE 3

Dr. Vimlesh Seth (VS)

Q.1. What does BCG stand for and how was it invented ?

BCG stands for Bacillus Calmette Guerin. It was prepared by Calmette & Guerin by repeated subcultures of Mycobacterium bovis on ox bile medium. Prior to its discovery, numerous investigators had tried to submit the tubercle bacilli to attenuate it, in order to produce a vaccine for the prevention of tuberculosis. In Lille(France), Albert Calmete (a bacteriologist) and Camille Guerin (a veterinarian) were working on the same with a highly virulent strain of tubercle bacilli of bovine origin, isolated a few years earlier by Nocard of Alfort from tuberculous mastitis in a heifer. In 1908, these workers observed that addition of beef bile, acting like a soap, melted the fatty surface of the bacilli and made possible the dissociation of the aggregates and their division almost to single units. The bacilli were then cultured & transplanted every three weeks for thirteen years (a total of 231 transplants). In 1921 the strain proved to be harmless even in highly susceptible guinea pigs; yet its antigenic properties were unimpaired. They called this bacillus, Bacillus Calmette & Guerin (BCG). In 1924 Calmette declared the bacillus incapable of reverting to virulent form. In 1928 the League of Nations declared the BCG strains as harmless in animals and man. Since then millions of infants and children have been BCG vaccinated all over the world.

Q.2. Why should BCG vaccine be given at left upper arm only ? Some parent insist that it should be given at gluteal region to avoid visible scar at the upper arm. Can BCG be given at sites other than left upper arm ?

It is a convention to give it on left upper arm, so that for take up of the vaccine, one is sure where to look for the scar.

B.C.G. vaccine should not be given at gluteal region, because the regional lymphadenitis there would prove to be more problematic. In any case, the scar of BCG is very small and produces no cosmetic problems. In some of the case it may even fade away completely.

Q.3. Why BCG ampoules are dark colored and so long in size while other vaccines (DPT, DT, Measles, MMT) are supplied in clear ampoules or vials ?

BCG ampoules, are dark colored because the vaccine deteriorates on exposure to light. A black paper is also usually supplied with each pack of BCG ampoules, to achieve the same objective.

The length of ampoule is kept long to avoid spillage of the powder while opening the ampoule.

Q.4. Are any special precautions necessary while opening a BCG ampoule and why ?

Ampoules of freeze dried BCG Vaccine are sealed under vacuum and there is no air or very little air in the ampoule. Thus they have to be opened carefully to avoid rushing in of air and spilling of powder.

The neck of the ampoule should not be crushed or broken suddenly by a metalic object. It should always be cut gradually at the junction of the neck and the body of the ampoule, by a cutter (file) so that air goes in slowly into the ampoule, and the powder is not spilled.

Q.5. BCG ampoules are supplied without any information regarding its dilution. Does this mean that any diluent can be used for its dilution ?

No, freeze dried BCG vaccine has to be reconstituted by dissolving it in normal saline as distilled water acts as an irritant to the skin. The diluent should always be kept with the vaccine in the main compartment of the refrigerator or in the cold box or in the vaccine carrier. It will ensure that it is cold enough when one needs it.

BCG is supplied as a 20 dose ampoule, it should be dissolved in 2 ml of normal saline. Vigorous shaking should not be done.

Q.6. For how long is the reconstituted dissolved vaccine potent ?

Reconstituted BCG vaccine should be used within 3 hours.

Q.7. Why do the manufacturers produce BCG in ampoules only ? Would it not be better if it is supplied in vials to avoid contamination of the diluted vaccine.

Once diluted, BCG has to be used within 3 hrs, so the question of keeping it safe for a longer period in a vial does not arise.

Q.8. How can the diluted vaccine be prevented from contamination ?

Contamination can be prevented as decided in the workshop on Immunization Practices in Children in 1988, as follows:

i) Seperate needle must be used for each child.

ii) Reconstitution of the ampoule should be done after washing hands and ensuring proper sterilization of equipment before proceeding for field work.

iii) syringes, needles and their box, forceps etc. are to be sterilized by boiling in water for 20 minutes.

iv) The red rubber rings and sections of rubber tubing meant for protection of vaccine from light is not to be boiled but should only be washed with soap and water. Open ampoule should be kept closed with a sterile cotton. contamination is unlikely to occur in 3 hours time.

Presently, it is far better to use disposable syringes and needles rather than to boil syringes and needles.

Q.9. Kindly tell us in which compartment of the refrigerator should we store BCG (undiluted and diluted) to maintain potency.

Diluted vaccine is not to be retained for more than 3-4 hours, hence storage is not required. However, undiluted vaccine should be stored in the middle of the main compartment. The temperature in this compartment is 2° to 4°C and at this temperalure freeze dried vaccine can be stored for upto 6 months. There is no need to put this vaccine in a freezer.

Q.10. An authentic study was conducted in Chingleput regarding the efficacy of BCG way back in 1980. It proved its ineffectiveness in preventing tuberculosis. But all the vaccination schedules still recommend BCG immunization.What do you have to say about it?

Reports from the tuberculosis prevention trial Chingleput, have been widely interpreted to show that BCG offers no protection against tuberculosis under any epidemiological conditions. This is not true as

i) The efficacy of BCG was assessed solely by the incidence of sputum positive pulmonary tuberculosis (Secondary or adult type).

ii) Extrapulmonary forms of tuberculosis, occuring in the study populations were not recorded

iii) Children under 10 years of age although vaccinated, were not included in the assessment lasting for seven and a half years.

iv) The report was written only seven and a half years after the beginning of the study and this period is not sufficient to study the natural history of tubercular infection.

The study had only shown the ineffectiveness of BCG vaccine to prevent adult type of tuberculosis and it is not justified to extrapolate these results to infants and children.

One must remember that even natural infection with tuberculosis does not protect against secondary type of tuberculosis and hence it would be futile to expect BCG (which provides much lesser immunity than natural infection) to do so.

The basic mechanism by which BCG acts, is by interfering with the silent bacillemia which follows after the very first exposure to human strain of tuberculous bacteria and hence it is most likely to be effective against hematogenous forms of primary tuberculosis. Other studies have shown that the incidence of hematogenous types of tuberculosis (the fatal form of tuberculosis) in infants and children is definitely lower in BCG vaccinated children. Also, some more studies from Thailand and Hongkong, done after Chingleput trial have also shown that the incidence of tuberculosis is lower in BCG vaccinated contacts of open case of tuberculosis. It is for all these reasons that BCG vaccine is still included in all immunization schedules.

Q.11. In several countries of the world (USA, UK) routine BCG is not given, still they have a low incidence of tuberculosis. Does this not mean that BCG has no role in eradicating tuberculosis ?

Yes, it is a fact that BCG is not given in UK and USA as a routine. It is because these countries have a very low incidence of tuberculosis and hence routine vaccination is not indicated in these countries. This is in conformity with the basic principle that vaccination is not required wherever the chances of natural infections are very low. This can not be interpreted to show that BCG is not helpful in controlling tuberculosis.

Q.12. Is there any decrease in the incidence of childhood tuberculosis in the last 10 years since EPI has been started? (especially whether there is decline of TBM or not)

There is a significant decrease in the incidence of childhood tuberculosis and specially TBM, as shown by Lotte et al, in Bas-Rhine data (1945-1984), as shown in Table-1.

Table 1

Age Specific Incidence of TB per 100,000.

Age gp(yrs)	*TB Cases*	*1965*	*70-74*	*75-79*	*80-84*
<5	*All forms*	*45.40*	*22.30*	*12.30*	*4.90*
	meningitis	*1.69*	*1.10*	*0.31*	*nil*
5-14	*All forms*	*36.70*	*15.00*	*7.60*	*6.90*
	meningitis	*0.82*	*0.14*	*0.14*	*0.15*
>5	*All forms*	*102.10*	*91.40*	*54.10*	*39.60*
	meningitis	*1.10*	*0.49*	*0.35*	*0.47*

BCG has been in use in India since 1953. Its use has been stepped up since 1978 with the introduction of EPI. However, it is difficult to say about its impact on tuberculosis prevalence in our country. Reliable estimates are difficult to come by, but it is generally estimated that there are 8 to 10 million cases of tuberculosis in India and 1 to 2 million cases are added every year. Reported incidence as given by Central Health Intelligence Bureau, Govt. of India has not shown any decline over the last 10 years. Regarding the incidence of TBM, again no reliable estimates are available but figures from LNJP hospital suggests that there has been a marginal decline in cases of TBM in 1984-1987 compared to 1955-58 period (1.8% vs 2.2% of all admissions).

Q.13. In UK, the BCG vaccine is given only at 12-13 year of age, while in India we give it at birth. Why is it so ?

BCG vaccination policy chosen for a particular area depends on its epidemiologic picture as suggested by WHO, ICMR study group. Thus, in areas of high prevalence, BCG should be given as early in life as possible, as the chances of a child acquiring infection early in life is very high. Thus, it is in early life only that the vaccine will have the greatest impact on serious sequelae of primary infection. In general, where more than 5% of children aged 10-14 years have been infected, BCG should be given at birth; where the rate is more than 2% but less than 5%, it should be given at school entry; and in places where less than 2% of children are infected at 10-14 years, BCG could be given at 12-13 years, thus affording maximum protection over the years of puberty. UK falls in the last category.

It seems that maximum BCG efficacy is seen within 1-2 years of vaccination and hence giving it just prior to the age when natural infection is most likely to occur in a given population is the most cost effective way of giving vaccine.

Q.14. There is a lot of confusion regarding the optimal age of vaccination. Some recommend at birth, while many others recommend at the age of one month. Recently, it is being recommended to be given between 3 and 9 month of age. Please clarify.

Although some studies have shown a slightly higher tuberculin conversion rate when BCG is given at 3 months of age, most studies have shown good sensitisation even when BCG was given at birth. Therefore, the current practice of giving BCG at birth is to be continued especially in view of the high endemicity of the disease in our country, and because it is so much easier to get the children at birth rather than at 1 or 3 months on a nation wide scale. If BCG has been missed at birth, then it should be given at the earliest contact, preferably before 9 months of age.

Q.15. BCG at birth may not produce any immunity. Is this true ?

This is not true. It has been shown that cell mediated immune response (CMIR) could be induced in a comparable proportion of cases at birth (78.2%) and at 3 months of age (72.5%). It is, therefore, considered that new borns are capable of evoking CMIR at birth and the practice of giving BCG at birth should be continued.

Q.16. Can preterm babies be vaccinated at birth? If so, is there any point (gestational age) below which vaccination is contraindicated?

BCG has been found to be effective in preterm infants also. Dawodu et al (1985) showed a tuberculin conversion rate of 83% in a group of preterm, appropriate for gestational age newborns (32-36 wks). However, small for gestational age babies have a poor tuberculin conversion following BCG vaccination.

Q.17. Similarly, is there any cut off point regarding birth weight and BCG vaccination ?

No specific references are available, but probably appropriate for gestational age 32-36 weeks newborns, may be treated as cut off. Babies above 2000 gm. can be easily vaccinated but it may be advisable to wait for some time for babies with lesser birth weight.

Q.18. I am unable to give intradermal injection. Can I give it by subcutaneous or intramuscular route? Can BCG be given orally?

No. BCG can not be given by subcutaneous or intramuscular route. Small abscesses are most likely to occur if the vaccine is given subcutaneously and the efficacy would be reduced.

Oral vaccination was used in France when BCG was first given and then in Brazil. A large dose of vaccine is required and must be followed by a milk feed to prevent cervical adenitis. The method is not advisable. Presently available vaccine cannot be used for oral use.

At present, there is no substitute for intradermal injection for BCG and the technique must be mastered by all those who wish to give BCG vaccination. 26 gauge needle should be used for giving intradermal injection.

Q.19. How should the skin be cleaned before giving BCG? Can spirit be used for this purpose?

No special preparation of the skin is necessary before giving BCG vaccination i.e. washing with disinfectants like alcohol, dettol etc. is not to be done. In fact, their use is contraindicated as they may destroy vaccine bacillus and thus affect the immune response adversely Cleaning with sterile water is enough.

Q.20. The method of using the same needle (after flaming) for BCG intradermal injection should be recommended or not? Can same syringe with only change of needles be advocated?

In mass campaigns, the needle is often passed through a naked flame for its sterilization. The organisms contained in the length of the needle are killed. This practice is to be strongly condemned and use of separate disposable or reusable autoclaved needles, must be adhered to for every case. The same syringe can however be used.

Q.21. How do I know that BCG has been given intradermally?

Raising a wheal over the injection site is a sure sign of intradermal injection. When an intradermal injection is given, hair follicles are seen as small pits on the wheal produced. This wheal should be clearly seen for all intradermal injections. When correct volume (0.1 cc) of vaccine is injected the wheal produced has a diameter of about 8mm.

Q.22. What is the dose of BCG vaccine? Does it vary with the age or weight of the child?

The standard dose of BCG vaccine is 0.1 mg in 0.1 ml volume, irrespective of age and weight of the child. The recommendation of reduced dose (0.05 mg in 0.05ml) in the first month of life is without any scientific explanation. A fear has been expressed by some workers that the rates of regional lymphadenitis are higher when higher dose (0.1mg) is given in infants. In controlled trials the incidence was 1.3% as compared to 1% with low dose (not a significant difference). Further, we are not sure of the efficacy of the lower dose of vaccine. Hence the same dose (i.e. 0.1mg) should be given at all the ages.

Q.23. Is rubbing at injection site of BCG, recommended soon after administration?

No, it is not desirable to disperse the bacteria contained in the vaccine from the intradermal site, otherwise the efficacy would be compromised. The wheal produced by BCG is not painful and would settle down in 20-30 minutes.

Q.24. I have given BCG today. What should I tell the mother who asked me whether she can bathe the child today?

Since the wheal settles in 20-30 minutes after vaccination, the mother can bathe the child the same day.

Q.25. Should hot fomentation be done at the injection site?

Though direct references are not available (in the case of BCG), actions and substances which increase local vascularity(such as rubbing, histamine, hyaluronidase etc) diminish the immune response. The same might hold true for formentation and hence it is not recommended.

Q.26. Do I need to give any other instructions to a mother of a baby who has received BCG today?

It is advisable to explain the expected reactions of vaccination to the mother in simplified language. The raised area will be absorbed in 20-30 minutes and would disappear and nothing will be seen at the site of injection for some days. By about the 3rd or 4th week, an area of hardness will be felt at the site of vaccination, which will become a lump of 6-10 mm by about the 6th week. It is generally not painful but may be tender to touch. The lump sometimes softens with pus formation which may discharge, leaving a tiny ulcer which heals by itself. After 10-12 weeks all that is visible is a tiny scar, 5-7 mm size, with a little pigmentation at the site. The process of healing and ulceration may repeat 2-3 times over a period of 2-3 months.

Q.27. Accidentally, I have injected 0.4 cc instead of 0.1 cc of BCG injection. What complications are anticipated?

Reactions to overdosage vary, from no recorded complications to local and nodal abscesses. In Britain, in one study, a group of children given a large overdose were immediately treated with INH for 60 days. No complications occurred. Hence, INH therapy may be indicated in a large accidental overdosage of BCG.

Practically it is impossible to give 0.4ml of BCG intradermally. If it has been injected, it has probably gone subcutaneous. The chances of local complications like abscess formation and suppurative lymphadenitis, increase with higher doses of BCG and with subcutaneous injection. It would be preferable to wait for any complication to occur, and then if required, to give INH therapy for 3-6 months. It may not be advisable to give INH right at the time of overdose injection, as it may interfere with the viability of injected bacilli and hence may interfere with the immune response.

Q.28. How long after BCG inoculation does Mantoux test become positive?

Taking responses of 5-6 mm as 'converted' in the case of newborns, 90% of the conversions will have occurred by six weeks, and 95% by 12 weeks.

Q.29. There is no indication of BCG take up even after 8 weeks of inoculation. Is there any recommendation for repeating BCG vaccination? If so, how long after this first BCG?

If no reaction is seen at the local site even after 12 weeks, it is an indication that BCG has not taken up. In such cases, BCG should be given again.

Q.30. Should Mantoux test be done in such a case before giving the second dose of BCG?

Yes, it would be preferable to give a Mantoux test in such children. If no reaction (≥5mm) is seen with ITU tuberculin even after 12 weeks of vaccination, then only the BCG vaccine may be given. Although it should be remembered that absence of reaction to Mantoux test does not necessarily mean that a hypersensitivity or immunity to tuberculosis has not been set up. In fact many of these children (i.e. Mx negative even after BCG) show a positive reaction to more sensitive tests of cell mediated immunity like phytehemaglutinin test (PHA) or lymphocyte migration inhibition test (LMIT).

Q.31. If there is no take up (reaction) after BCG vaccination, then what are the reasons for it? Is the vaccine not potent or the technique faulty?

Either of the factors i.e. the potency of BCG and faulty technique, may be operative when no reaction to BCG is obtained. If the instructions regarding storage, transport etc. are not followed meticulously, the vaccine may be inactivated. If the vaccine is given subcutaneously, it may not evoke adequate cell mediated immune response, and also if adequate dose is not given the vaccine may not take up. Apart from potency of BCG and the technique, certain host factors (like malnutrition, measles etc) may also interfere with uptake of BCG.

Q.32. Reaction to BCG has appeared after 4 days of inoculation (instead of 4 weeks). What can be the cause of it?

This is an accelerated response to BCG, popularly known as positive BCG test. Like tuberculin test it indicates that this subject has had exposure to tubercular infection or vaccine (BCG) and needs investigations for the same.

Contrary to the claims of some research workers, an accelerated BCG reaction is not suggestive of active tuberculosis. It is probably not desirable to use BCG test routinely but to reserve it only for severly ill, malnourished and Mantou negative individuals. It should also be remembered that apparently accelerated reaction may often be due to contaminated vaccine.

Q.33. Is there any need for booster dose (revaccination) after some years? For how long BCG immunity normally lasts?

Tuberculin hypersensitivity after BCG vaccination is known to wane over a period of time. Thus only 34% of children are still LMIT positive after 5 years of BCG vaccination. Further, it has also been observed that BCG given at birth is not protective against adult type of tuberculosis. These factors suggest the need for revaccination with BCG.

Revaccination with BCG at 6-8 years and again at 11-14 years in Romania, has been shown to be helpful in decreasing the incidence of late childhood and adult type of tuberculosis. Many countries in SE Asia are routinely using revaccination in their National Health Programmes. WHO, on the other hand does not recommend revaccination. Although, by and large there is no consensus on revaccination with BCG but it may be considered in Mantoux negative 5 year old children.

Q.34. Should Mantoux test be done prior to BCG vaccination in older children. Till what age BCG can be given without performing a mantoux test?

In office practice, it is preferable to do Mantoux testing before giving BCG in all age groups except in children below 1 year of age in whom BCG can be given without Mantoux testing.

Q.35. National Tuberculosis Control Programme recommends giving BCG even in older children without prior Mantoux testing. This is contrary to what I was taught. What is you opinion?

In a tuberculin test survey done over a period of 5 years, it was realised that in an mass immunization programme, as also in large number of children attending outpatient services, the drop out rate is 51% if we decide to do BCG vaccination after tuberculin testing. Thus, there was enormous waste of hospital time. Tuberculin test could not be read in 51% cases. The dropout rate from Nagpur data was as high as 74.83% Thus, such a procedure though ideal, would be futile and impractical at a field level. Since the studies were conducted in 0-14 years age group, no cut off point for tuberculin test prior to B.C.G. is recommended, in the national health programme.

Direct BCG vaccination of even previously exposed (Mx+ve) children does not cause any adverse reactions except an accelerated reaction and hence is quite safe.

Q.36. A newborn is born to a mother who is an open case of tuberculosis (TB). How can he be protected from TB. Can such a mother breast feed her child? Can BCG and antituberculous treatment (ATT) be given together.

A rational approach would consist of

i) Treatment of the mother, and

ii) Protection of the newborn.

i) **Treatment of the mother**: The mother of such a newborn has to be treated intensively with 3 or 4 drugs. There is no need to isolate the infant from the mother. It has been demonstrated that INH administered to newborns prevented infection even when the infants remained with their mothers, suffering from open tuberculosis. Breast feeding is not contraindicated as the infection does not spread through breast milk and would be preferable over bottle feeding as in any other child. None of the antitubercular drugs are excreted in sufficient amounts in breast milk to cause any toxicity to the newborn.

ii) **Protection of the newborns**: All the newborns born to infectious mothers, should be put on INH (10mg/kg) prophylaxis after excluding congenital tuberculosis. They should be observed clinically over the next 3 months, if any symptom like failure to thrive, fever etc. develop, the child should be screened for tuberculosis and treated for the same with 3-4 drugs. If the child remains healthy, a Mantoux test should be given at 3 months. If it is negative, BCG is given and INH is stopped. But if Mantoux at 3 months is positive, child is investigated for tuberculosis and treated appropriately with 2 or 3 drugs for one year.

Q.37. Is INH resistant BCG available which can be used concurrently with INH administration to prevent TB?

Routinely available BCG cannot be given simultaneously with antitubercular treatment. INH resistant BCG has been developed and found to be equally effective as ordinary BCG. This is not yet available in India.

Some workers have suggested that even routinely available BCG can be given with INH with equal efficacy. The plan outlined above (Q36) obviates the need of INH resistant BCG.

Q.38. A child has already been treated for tuberculosis. Does this child need BCG ?

The fundamental purpose of BCG is to give a non-pathogenic primary infection, using a measured dose of an attenuated bovine mycobacterium. The primary infection induces tuberculin hyper-sensitivity and increases defence mechanisms so that if the recipient is later exposed to reinfection with a pathogenic strain of mycobacteria, that infection will not cause a clinical disease or if it does, then it will be localized. In other words, once tuberculized naturally, the child already has primary infection and hence would not need BCG.

Q.39. Is this not a idea to give BCG to all children who are Mantoux positive to protect them from flaring up of tuberculosis. In other words can BCG protect against recrudescence type of secondary tuberculosis?

Mantoux positivity indicates that the person has been exposed to tuberculosis and has acquired at least primary infection (clinical or subclinical). Thus, going by the analogy mentioned in previous question, the role expected to be filled by BCG has already been achieved. There is thus no need of giving BCG to such children. BCG prevents bacteremia following primary infection with *Mycobacterium tuberculosis.*

There is no evidence till now that it can help in preventing recrudescence type of tuberculosis. Further, BCG in a Mantoux positive child tends to produce an accelerated reaction with an increased incidence of local lymphadenitis.

Q.40. Can BCG vaccine be given along with measles vaccine?

Ideally different live vaccines should not be given at the same time. A period of 4-6 weeks should elapse before the next vaccination is given.

It is preferable not to give these two vaccines together., Measles vaccine is known to depress cell mediated immunity. This may therefore interfere with the uptake of BCG. A 6 weeks gap should be there between measles vaccine and BCG.

Q.41. Which vaccines can be given concurrently with BCG and which vaccines should not be given simultaneously with BCG ?

BCG can be given with OPV or DPT at the same time. Measles and MMR should not be given with BCG.

Q.42. I try to avoid giving two injections to children on one visit. For example a two months old child is brought to me for vaccination. I give BCG at first visit and tell them to come after few days for DPT and Polio vaccination. Parents accept this practice. do you agree with me ?

There is no harm in giving DPT and Polio on the same day as BCG, but if for some reason, they are not given on the same day, then a gap of at least 4 weeks must elapse between two vaccinations. A lesser gap will interfere with the uptake of both BCG, DPT and Polio.

Q.43. An ulcer has formed at BCG inoculation site. It is not healing even after 8 weeks. Which antibiotics (local/parenteral) do you recommend to treat this condition? What is the suggested management?

Ulcer formation at BCG inoculation site is a normal phenomenon. The phenomenon of healing and ulceration may repeat 2-3 times over a period of 8-12 weeks. Nothing needs to be done for this. Antibiotics are not needed unless there is evidence of secondary infection like cellulitis or abscess formation. In these cases erythromycin would be the drug of choice.

Q.44. Can ATT be tried in this case of nonhealing ulcer?

ATT is not required for the so called non healing ulcer. Almost all of these ulcers would heal spontaneously within 4-5 months of vaccination.

Q.45. Following BCG, an axillary lymph node has formed. What should be done?

Local lymph node enlargement is also a normal component of BCG uptake, suggesting formation of a primary complex. Nothing needs to be done for this if the lymph node is less than 1.5 cm in size and is not suppurating. ATT in the form of only INH (10mg/kg/day) for 3 months would be required if either the gland is progressively increasing in size or if it shows signs of suppuration. Excision may be required in an occasional case where a sinus formation is threatened.

Q.46. Can neck glands also enlarge in response to BCG infection?

Yes, if BCG vaccination is given high up on the shoulder, the bacilli reach the nodes in supra clavicular or anterior triangle of the neck.

Q.47. I get a chest X-ray done on a 4 year old child to rule out tuberculosis. Left axilla shows calcified glands. Can this be due to BCG vaccination given in infancy or this may be due to tuberculosis?

Calcified left axillary gland is generally due to BCG vaccination. Primary infection of the lung leads to either hilar or paratracheal calcification .

Q.48. A 2 year old child has been brought with history of definite BCG vaccination at birth but there is no scar. What should be done?

Absence of scar, despite definite BCG vaccination, in a 2 year old child suggests that the child had failed to react to the vaccination. Although theoretically, a scar once formed can also disappear (See Q.490) but it is too early to do so by 2 years. Revaccination should be considered if the child does not react to a test dose of tuberculin (≥ 6 mm to 1 TU)

Q.49. In a 8 years old child there is no BCG scar. According to the parents a scar was present initially and now it has faded. Is it possible? If so, does it mean that the immunity has also decreased? What should be done in such a case ?

Yes, BCG scars are known to disappear over a period of time, but the disappearance of scar is not synonymous with either decrease of hypersensitivity or immunity. Nevertheless revaccination should be done if child does not react to a test dose of tuberculin (≥ 6 mm to 1 TU).

Q.50. A 5 year old child with a positive BCG scar, is being investigated for tuberculosis. His Mantoux test is negative and the rest of the investigations are also normal. Having excluded tuberculosis, do I need to give BCG to this child again as his Mantoux is negative ?

Opinion on this may differ. It is well known that LMIT may still be positive when the Mantoux has become negative, thus suggesting that hypersensitivity to BCG still persists. Nevertheless most authorities would now recommend giving BCG to such children. It may be better to test with a higher strength (5TU) tuberculin before giving BCG to such children.

It should be remembered that revaccination with BCG may lead to an accelerated reaction in this individual. This should not be interpreted as positive BCG test.

Q.51. Can BCG be administered concurrently with Mantoux test at the same sitting. Is Mantoux reaction affected by BCG administration ?

Yes, they can be given but there is no justification for such a procedure. Mantoux given on the same day as

BCG is not going to be affected by it. Mantoux test becomes positive only after 6-8 weeks of BCG administration.

Q.52. BCG is used by some in the diagnosis of tuberculosis. Do you recommend such a practice ?

The diagnostic use of BCG has been recommended as BCG has a higher positivity rate compared to mantoux test, in proven/suspected and malnourished cases of tuberculosis. The BCG injection evokes various types of reactions like, classical, accelerated, delayed, complete or incomplete. They all have varying significance in TB diagnosis and are much more informative than Mantoux test alone.

BCG has been shown to be more sensitive in evoking hypersensitivity reactions in persons exposed to tuberculosis, esp. those in suffering with malnutrition or with disseminated diseases. However it should be remembered that even increasing dose of tuberculin in Mantoux test (from 1 to 10 to 100 TU), progressively evokes more positive reactions, many of which be falsely positive.

A strength of 1 TU or 5 TU tuberculin is recommended for Mantoux testing, only to avoid these false positive reactions. Although Udani has tried to distinguish various types of reactions following BCG test, the criteria applied and the interpretations of the same are rather subjective and prone to misinterpretations. Further, BCG vaccine (even when given as test) will interfere with further Mantoux testing also. Thus, we consider the routine use of BCG test in office practice as totally unwarranted and harmful. It may be occasionally considered in hospitalised, severely malnourished, Mantoux negative children who are strongly suspected to have tuberculosis.

Q.53. I gave BCG to a nine months old child who developed measles after 10 days of inoculation. What should be done ?

Isoniazide chemoprophylaxis in a dose of 10 mg/kg/day during risk period (for 12 weeks following measles infection) is to be administered to children who develop measles or whooping cough within 4-6 weeks of BCG administration, to prevent possible dissemination.

It will be advisable to ensure Mantoux conversion in such children as BCG may not take up in such circumstances.

Q.54. Can BCG be given to children who are on long term steroids or chemotherapy (i.e. compromised hosts) ?

No. They are at increased risk of disseminated tuberculosis if BCG is given. A minimum period of 6-8 weeks must elapse after stopping steroids before giving BCG.

Q.55. Can BCG be given to a child who has received immunoglobulin 10 days back?

It is best avoided for another 4 weeks.

Although it is generally agreed that cell mediated immunity is the major component of immune reaction with BCG, recently it has been shown that even humoral immunity also plays an important part in preventing tubercular infection. Therefore it is theoretically possible that BCG may be affected after immunoglobulin administration. It would be advisable therefore to postpone BCG for 4-6 weeks. If given earlier, it should be ensured that BCG has been successfully taken up by demonstrating a Mantoux conversion.

Q.56. Can BCG be given to children with congenital infections (TORCH)?

BCG efficacy has been in doubt in low birth weight neonates with severe intrauterine growth retardation who weigh less than 3rd percentile for their gestational age. These factors and accompanying secondary immunosuppression are often found co-existing in children with congenital infections. Immunization would depend on the presence/absence and interplay/severity of these factors and in general BCG should be avoided in these neonates.

Q.57. Can BCG be given to a child with hepatitis B infection ?

In general, all viral infections have an effect on the immune response of an individual which may differ from virus to virus. BCG status in all these infections has not been worked out. Hence it is best to avoid BCG for a period of 4-6 weeks following a viral infection. An exception to this statement would be hepatitis B. BCG is a nonspecific stimulator of cell mediated immunity and therefore BCG vaccination may be helpful as an immunomodulator in chronic hepatitis B infection.

Q.58. Can BCG be given to a child with chicken pox whose skin lesions have already dried up ?

There is no definite data on this. It is not known whether there are any immunological changes following chicken pox infection but like all other viral infections, it will be preferable to wait for 4-6 weeks.

Q.59. How soon BCG be given to a child after an attack of measles ?

BCG can be given anytime after 12 weeks of measles infection.

Q.60. Can BCG cause tuberculous disease? If so, under what conditions ?

BCG can cause tuberculous disease dissemination in following conditions:

i) Immuno deficiency states.

ii) Incubation period of another infection particularly measles.

iii) Sometime soon after birth in small for dates.

Q.61. Why BCG cannot be made available in single dose ampoules ?

Single dose ampoules will not be cost effective in countries like India where mass BCG vaccination strategy is implemented. Also, since the same syringe can be used with change of needles for different people, waste incurred is hardly any.

The size of BCG ampoule has been made for mass campaigns. In office practice wastage can be minimised if a separate day (once in a week/fortnight/month) is kept for BCG vaccination. Of course, it would be still better if smaller ampoules can be provided for office practice.

Q.62. As per government instructions, no child should be denied any vaccination and ampoule of vaccine is to be opened even for a single child. What are your comments ? Will it not lead to a lot of wastage ?

Cost of a wasted ampoule will always be less than that of a full course of anti-tubercular therapy which might be needed if immunization is withheld and the child develops active disease.

Bibliography

1. BCG vaccination. In manual of Immunization, Department of Family Planning, Kotla Road, New Delhi pp. 18-25.
2. Dawodu AH. Tuberculin conversion following BCG vaccination in preterm infants. Acta Paediatr Scand. 1985, 74: 564-67.
3. Editorial. BCG vaccination of humans: In: Advances in Tuberculosis Research Vol 22 DW Smith & Karger 1985. pp 29-30.

4. Immunization Programme. Manual for health workers, Ministry of Health and Family Welfare. Govt. of India, New Delhi 1986.
5. Kathipari K, Seth V et al.: Cell mediated immune response after BCG as a determinant optimum age of vaccination. Ind J Med Res. 1982, 76: 508-571.
6. Lote et al. Second IUATLD study on complications in intradernal BCG vaccination. Bulletin International Union Against Tuberculosis 1988, 63: 49-56.
7. Mehta R. Mittal SK & Saini L. BCG test applications in Pediatric Practice. Ind Pediatr 1986, 23: 419-428
8. Menon MPS, BCG vaccine, in: Pulmonary Tuberculosis. National Book Trust, New Delhi, India 1987, pp 223, 229.
9. Miller FJW. BCG vaccination, In: TB in children. Churchil Livingstone 1982, pp. 55-63
10. Mittal SK and Gupta RC Falacy of BCG test. Ind Pediatric 1981, 18:680.
11. Seth V. et al. CMIR at varying age periods in relation to the nutritional status among preschool children given BCG at birth. J Trop Pediatr 1984, 30: 210-213.
12. Seth V et al: Persistence of *in vitro* lymphocyte response to tuberculin, in skin test negative children immunised with BCG in infancy. Acta paediatr. Scand. 1977, 66: 569-573.
13. Seth V. Antituberculous therapy in children. Ind J Pediat. 1986, 53: 179-188.
14. Sethi GR, B.C.G. In Immunisation Practices in Children. Editors AK Dutta, SK Mittal & V Agarwal I.AP., Delhi, 1988 p. 1-7.
15. Udani P.M. : Evaluation of Tuberculin Test in Pediatric Practice. Ind Pediatr 1982, 19: 469-486.
16. Udani P.M. : BCG test in tuberculosis. Ind Pediatr 1971, 8: 143-150.
17. Udani P.M. Is Booster dose of BCG Vaccine necessary ? Ind J Pediatr. 1989: 56, 311-320.

DPT VACCINE

1. **Contents:** Each 0.5 ml contains:
   Diphtheria toxoid 25 Lf
   Tetanus toxoid 5 Lf.
   Pertussis 4 I.U. (20,000 million killed bacteria)
2. **Ideal age of initiating primary vaccination:**
   6 to 8 weeks
3. **Schedule of primary vaccination:**
   Three doses at 4-8 weeks interval.
4. **Boosters:** Two at 1.5 years & 4-5 years.
5. **When recommended:** Routine Immunization.
6. **Dose :** 0.5ml.
7. **Route of administration**: Deep intramuscular.
8. **Site of administration**: Anterolateral aspect of thigh.
9. **Preparation of site of administration**: Clean with spirit.
10. **Instructions to the mother after vaccination:**
    To give antipyretic (paracetamol) in case of fever.
11. **Protection/efficacy :**
    Pertussis - 80%, Diphtheria and Tetanus almost 100%
12. **Contra-indications**
    a. Progressive neurological disease.
    b. Uncontrolled convulsions.
    c. Severe reactions to first or subsequent dose.
13. **Side effects**: Fever, local pain.
14. **Complications:**
    Convulsions, screaming episodes, shock, encephalitis.
15. **Storage at different levels and at doctor's clinic:**
    a) **When the vaccine is not use:**
       In lower most compartment of fridge (Do not freeze)
    b) **During immunization session:**
       Can be kept at room temperature.
    c) **In case of electricity failure:** Keep at cool & dark place.

D P T VACCINE 4

Dr. Lata Kumar (LK) & Dr. A.K. Dutta (AKD)

Q.1. Is no uniformity required regarding the composition of DPT in our country ? Is there any need to do something about it ?

There is a definite need for uniformity in the composition of DPT vaccine. The vaccines produced in India now a days are more or less uniform and are within the prescribed limits of the National Pharmacopia. Commonly available vaccines in India at present contain 25 LF of DT, 5 LF of T.T. and 4 I.U. (Equivalent to 20,000 million killed bacteria) of pertussis per dose.

W.H.O. has recently suggested that the vaccine may be standardised as per its potency rather than by its content. It suggests that each vaccine dose should have a potency of 4,30, and 40 I.U. of pertussis and diphtheria, and tetanus toxoid respectively. This procedure has not yet been introduced in our countiy but by and large the L.F. content of diphtheria and tetanus toxoid, in the available vaccines, has the required potency.

Q.2. Different manufacturers make DPT of varying constitutions. Which one do you prefer ?

Till a few years ago there were differences in the content of DPT vaccine as manufactured by different pharmaceuticals. At present, however, this situation has been remedied and now all vaccines manufactured in our country have the same amounts of different antigens. Hence any one of them can be used with equal effectiveness.

Q.3. What is the efficacy of DPT injections ?

If DPT vaccination is given at the proper times and at right intervals, then more than 80% efficacy has been observed against pertussis. The efficacy is over 95% against diphtheria and tetanus.

Q.4. The first dose of DPT is being recommended at 6 weeks of age. What is the basis of this? Is it better than giving at 12 weeks of age ? Can we start even earlier than this ?

LK : DPT is recommended at 6 weeks of age because the mother is called at 6 weeks for postnatal check up. It is convenient to give it at the time the mother also comes. This reduces one visit by the mother. Scientifically, there is no significant difference in giving Ist dose at 6 weeks or at 12 weeks of age.

AKD : Transfer of maternal antibody against pertussis, diphtheria & tetanus is uncommon and most women of child bearing age lack demonstrable antibodies. As a result passive immunity during early infancy is uncommon and whooping cough may develop soon after birth. The case fatality rate at this age is very high. Early immunization therefore is important. Active immunization of the mother with tetanus toxoid during pregnancy helps to prevent neonatal tetanus. But such a procedure cannot be adopted for whooping cough & diphtheria, as these antigens are not well tolerated in adults.

Almost all studies have shown that pertussis vaccine aministration before the age of 4 weeks does not produce significant antibody response. Most studies have shown that seroconversions are uniformly satisfactory when the pertussis vaccination is started at any time after 8 weeks of age. There are not enough studies for seroconversion at 6 weeks but the available studies suggest that adequate seroconversion can be obtained even when the pertussis vaccination is started at that age. Keeping in mind the need for early immunisation against whooping cough (and also probably against polio) the WHO Global Advisory Committee on E.P.I. suggested shifting of age of vaccination to 6 weeks instead of 12 weeks.

It may be noted here that Diphtheria and Tetanus toxoids as such are quite effective even in the first week of life. Also these are excellent antigens and even two doses given at 4 weeks interval irrespective of the age of initiation, usually give adequate seroconversion, but difficulties are encountered with pertussis vaccine. Probably the best results are obtained when the first two doses are given at 8 week interval and the 3rd dose is delayed for 6 months after the second dose, as practised in UK. This even obviates the need for a booster at 18 months. But this schedule is not practical in a national health programme because of the need to combine this with OPV and also because it would lead to large number of drop outs. 3 doses of pertussis starting at 3 months given at 4 weeks interval give about 80% pretection. None of the studies in recent times (except one in 1949) has actually studied the immunological efficacy of present day schedule i.e. 6, 10 & 14 weeks but extrapolation of data from various studies employing 3 dose schedule, suggest that it may be sufficiently effective.

Q.5. What is the ideal interval between the primary doses of DPT ? What is the scientific basis for the spacing of 3 primary DPT doses ?

The best response of DPT vaccine is seen when the interval is 8 weeks or more. However, it has been observed that in countries where there is a risk of the disease in early infancy and if the interval is made 8 weeks, there is increased risk of the disease occurring in the susceptible individuals, even before the schedule can be completed. Moreover there is a feeling that there is an increase in drop out rates if 8 weeks interval is recommended. The seroconversion studies conducted following 4 weeks interval showed that the antibody response was little less initially but the final immunity is not altered and remains the same.

Q.6. If first dose of DPT is given at the right time i.e. at 6 weeks of age and there is a lapse of more than 6 months for the second dose, is

there any need for restarting the series once again or only second then third dose is to be given ?

There is no need to restart the series of D.P.T. vaccine if any of the vaccine doses is missed, irrespective of the lapsed interval, as the immunological memory once induced is never lost. Only the remaining doses i.e. 2nd and 3rd doses are to be given.

Q.7. **First and second dose of DPT were given at the right time. For the third dose the child had reported at the age of 1 year. What should be done ?**

The third dose should be given, as explained earlier.

Q.8. **An infant comes to us at 1-1/2 Years of age. He had received two primary doses of DPT at the age of 4 and 5 months respectively. Should the third dose of DPT or the booster dose be given in such a child ?**

Only one dose of DPT is to be given whether you call it a booster or the third dose.

Q.9. **What should be the minimum interval between third primary dose and first booster dose ? For example if an infant completes his three primary doses by 1-1/4 years of age then at what age should the first booster be given ?**

A booster given earlier than 6 months after the third primary dose fails to evoke adequate antibody response. This is because of the persistence of antibodies formed by primary vaccination which interfere with the uptake of the booster dose. After 6 month the antibodies induced by the last dose of primary series wane away sufficiently to allow a meaningful antibody response to the booster dose. This child should receive his booster at or after the age of 1 year 9 months.

Q.10. What site should be preferred for intramuscular injection of DPT to infants and older children ? After what age is the gluteal site preferred to the lateral aspect of thigh ?

The DPT vaccine should be given deep intramuscular. In infants lateral aspect of the thigh is to be preferred as it offers a safe area (free of nerves and vessels) with adequate muscle mass. Although outer and upper part of buttocks can be used after infancy, in actual practice it would probably still be safer to use lateral aspects of thigh even after that age.

Q.11. Why should DPT be given deep intramuscular injection ?

Deep intramuscular injection causes less local reaction.

Q.12. What will happen if some DPT is injected accidentally into the vein (while being injected deep I/M) ? Can this be avoided.

AKD : Yes, This should and can be avoided, provided an effort is made to draw the piston out while injecting, and to observe whether there is any blood in the syringe. However there is no specific case report of I.V. administration and it is difficult to predict the side effects.

L.K : Theoretically nothing should happen if small amounts are injected into the vein. However, immunity is unlikely to develop if the injection is given into the vein.

Q.13. Which antiseptic should be used for cleaning the site of injection ?

Any antiseptic, preferably spirit.

Q.14. Should vigorous rubbing be done at injection site soon after administration ?

No, it should be avoided.

Q.15. Do you recommend first dose of antipyretic to be given at the time of injection ?

No. Not routinely. Paracetamol (15mg/kg/dose) should be advised to be taken as and when the child has fever. It may be preferable to give paracetamol at the time of injection itself, to a child with personal or family history of convulsive disorders.

Q.16. Which antipyretic do you recommend for post DPT fever and pain ?

Paracetamol is the preferred drug. Use of aspirin, analgin or meftal is better avoided.

Q.17. A child has not been moving the injected right lower limb for 3 days since the DPT injection. What should be done ?

It is not uncommon to encounter this problem following DPT injection. This is due to the local pain and inflammation and is more likely to happen if the injection has not gone deep. This usually lasts for 2-3 days and requires only analgesics and hot fomentations. Rarely polio may be precipitated by the intramuscular injection (of any substance including DPT) and be the cause of this complain. This should be obvious on physical examination. Sciatic paralysis should be considered if the gluteal site is used for vaccination.

Q.18. A child has developed marked induration and pain at the injection site. Should antibiotics be given to treat this situation ? What else can be done ?

The induration and pain usually subsides by 2-3 days. If it persists for more than 3 days, cellulitis and abscess should be suspected and if it is proved, then antibiotics are indicated. Use of disposable syringes and needles will avoid such situations.

Q.19. A child had developed a painless residual nodule in the thigh as a result of DPT injection which was given 3 months back What should be done ?

Nothing needs to be done. This will dissolve in due course of time.

Q.20. Should first dose of DPT be delayed in preterms ?

Yes, he can be given the vaccine. There is no role of reduced dose of DPT, as this will not produce enough immunity.

Q.21. A 2 months old infant of 2 kg. weight has been brought to my office for first dose of DPT vaccination. Can this child be given DPT vaccination, should we wait till the weight is 3 Kg or should we give half the dose of DPT ?

Yes, he can be given the vaccine. There is no role of reduced dose of DPT, as this will not produce enough immunity.

A number of studies have suggested that a reduction in dosages of Diphtheria/Pertussis/Tetanus vaccine does not reduce the rate of local & systemic reaction. Although one study suggested efficacy with reduced dose, but this is somewhat controversial and can not be recommended.

Q.22. Is there a different schedule for vaccination of malnourished children ?

No, studies have clearly shown that even severely malnourished children are capable of adequate immunological response to DPT vaccine.

Q.23. What is ideal in day to day practice, DPT vials or DPT ampoules ?

It depends upon the number of infants you expect in one immunization session. Both are equally good.

Q.24. If we use the multiple dose vial can we use the left over vaccine in next vaccination session ?

Yes, if you can avoid contamination.

Q.25. Can BCG, DPT, and polio be administered simultaneously in case the infant has reported for the first time, say at the age of 2 months ?

Yes, there is no harm in giving these vaccines on the same day. This in fact will be preferable.

Q.26. Which other vaccines can simultaneously be administered with DPT & which vaccines can not be given ?

Any EPI vaccine except typhoid vaccine can be administered simultaneously with DPT but at separate sites.

Q.27. In which compartment of the refrigerator should DPT be stored ?

It should not be kept in the freezer compartment or in the door of the refrigerator. It can be kept in any other chamber.

It is usually recommended to be kept in the lower most chamber of the fridge.

Q.28. Accidentally the DPT vaccine got frozen in the refrigerator. Can I use this vaccine after rewarming ?

No, freezing and rewarming (thawing) destroys the vaccine.

Q.29. Few of the children do not get fever after DPT injection. Should the potency of vaccine be suspected in such cases ?

The incidence of febrile reaction following DPT is only 20-30%. So absence of fever is not an indication of poor potency.

Q.30. Is there any contraindication for the first dose of DPT ?

First dose of DPT is contraindicated only if there is a progressive neurological disorder in the child.

Q.31. A child of convulsive disorder is on regular doses of anticonvulsant. Can this child be given DPT, or should DT be given in such cases ?

DPT can be given if the child is already on anticonvulsants and the convulsions are well controlled. The child should receive antipyretics at the time of injection. DT is to be given if the seizures are not controlled.

Q.32. Can Children of cerebral palsy be given DPT injection?

Yes, remember cerebral palsy is a non-progressive disorder of motor function.

Q.33. A lot of reactions can occur due to DPT vaccine including shock like syndrome. Can we do sensitivity testing (like we do with pencillin) before giving the vaccine ?

No, because the shock like syndrome is extremely rare. In any case, subcutaneous injection (for sensitivity testing) with DPT is not to be given.

Q.34. Should 'precious' children be given DT instead of DPT (to avoid the possible adverse effects of DPT)?

Every child is precious, moreover, if the child is 'precious' there is more reason to give him DPT rather than DT. Remember the complications with pertussis vaccine are far less than those with natural disease.

Q.35. A two years old child has recovered from whooping cough. A primary series of vaccination is to be started. Should DPT or DT be given in such a case ?

A natural infection with pertussis does not ensure protection against future attacks of whooping cough. Therefore DPT should be given to this child. No adverse reactions are expected.

Q.36. A newborn is born to a mother who did not receive tetanus vaccination during pregnancy. Should the newborn be given tetanus immunoglobulin or tetanus toxoid for immediate protection against tetanus ?

It should not be a routine practice. However, TIG as well TT can be given at birth especially when delivery was conducted by untrained dai in unhygenic conditions.

The best method to prevent neonatal tetanus is by active immunisation of mother (by two injection of TT) during pregnancy. This ensures almost 100% protection and is absolutely safe. Aseptic care of the cord at the time of delivery and thereafter is of equal importance. TIG at birth may be given if aseptic care cannot be ensured. TT in any case will take minimum of 7-15 days to be effective and would not be of much help in preventing neonatal tetanus.

Q.37. A child suffered from convulsions after the first dose of DPT. Can second dose of DPT be given safely to this child or should DT be given in future in such cases ? Or should DPT be given under cover of anticonvulsants ?

Second and successive doses should be DT and not DPT

It is not advisable to give DPT even under cover of anticonvulsants.

Only convulsions occuring within 3 days of immunization, with or without fever should be considered to be due to DPT vaccine.

Q.38. A child became very sick (kept on screaming for 4 hours continuously) after first dose of DPT. What precautions should be used for the next dose of DPT ?

Second and successive doses should be DT, as the incidence of recurrence of persistent screaming is high if DPT is again given.

Q.39. Do serious reactions to DPT occur with first dose only or can they occur with subsequent doses also ? In other words if a child does not suffer from any untoward reactions with first dose of DPT then is this child unlikely to suffer from reactions to subsequent doses of DPT ?

The reactions can occur with any of the doses and not necessarily with the first dose only.

Q.40. What are the contraindications to second & successive doses of DPT ?

Second and successive doses of DPT are contraindicated if any of the following complications occur after the previous dose.

i) Convulsions.
ii) Encephalopathy.
iii) Anaphylaxis.
iv) Hyporesponsive or Hypotensive (shock like syndrome) episode.
v) Hyperpyrexia with fever, equal to or greater than 105°F.
vi) Persistent and high pitched crying for more than 3 hours.

Convulsions occuring within 72 hours and encephalopathy occuring within 7 days of DPT injection should be attributed to DPT vaccine and be considered as contraindication to further doses of DPT. This time frame is important if these reactions are to be considered to be due to DPT itself.

Q.41. If a child becomes very sick after DPT injection then what is the medico-legal position ?

If the child had significant reaction to an earlier dose, and becomes very sick following subsequent doses, or when the dose is given in face of absolute contraindication, the doctor is liable for legal action.

Unpredictable reactions to first dose can occur even in the absence of progressive neurological disease. In such cases, although the doctor may still be taken to court, legally he cannot be held responsible for the adverse reaction.

Q.42. A child has suffered from encephalopathy following DPT vaccination. Should DPT be given or not to the younger sibling ? Is there any genetic predisposition to adverse reactions ?

DPT can be safely given to the younger sibling of the child who developed encephalopathy following DPT vaccination as there is no known genetic predisposition to adverse reactions.

Q.43. What is the critical age beyond which DPT should not be given and only DT be given ?

At present pertussis component of the DPT is not recommended after 6-7 years of age. However, in the recent international symposium on pertussis immunization, there has been a suggestion that pertussis component can be given even to adults without significant adverse reactions.

No doubt adults can be given, but they should not be given, for the simple reason that they don't need it. Also remember that reactions to Diphtheria toxoid (in full dose) are very severe in older children and adults.

Q.44. If after 2 years of age primary immunization is to be started then how many doses of DPT/DT should be given. And what about booster doses ?

If the child has come before 4 years of age, 3 doses of DPT should be given as usual, followed by one booster after 3 yrs of first booster if the child is still below 6 years of age. If the child is more than 6 years of age then two primary doses of DT and one booster needs to be given.

Q.45. A child has received first booster of DPT at the age of 3 years when should the second booster be given ?

Second booster is to be given at the appropriate time of the schedule i.e. at 5 yrs of age.

Q.46. A child has received his second booster of DPT today (at 4.5 years of age). when should I call him next ?

He should be recalled at 10 years of age for a dose of Td and thereafter every 10 years for TT vaccine.

He may also need to be called for typhoid vaccine every 3 years or so.

Q.47. What is the difference in the immunity status at the age of 1 year between 2 infants, if one has received a regular course of primary DPT (6 weeks - 10 weeks - 14 weeks) while another received irregular course of DPT (2 months, 7 months and 10 months) ?

Final immunity will be the same. Only difference is that when irregular schedule is being practiced e.g. 2 months, 7 months and 10 months, the infant remains susceptible during the period of 2 to 7 months, as one dose is not sufficient to protect the individual.

Q.48. Why is DT being recommended as second booster instead of DPT in recent schedules ?

There is no clear cut data or any study done in our country to omit 2nd booster of DPT. Available evidence still suggests that the 2nd booster dose of DPT must be given at 4-5 years of age. If the dose is omitted, the child becomes susceptible to develop the disease at an older age, i.e. after 6 years of age. He will then become an important source of infection to other children.

Although the case fatality rate of pertussis is highest under 1 year of age, the maximum incidence of pertussis is seen between 5-9 years of age. These children are a great source of infection in the community including the younger siblings at home. Further, antibody levels, after first booster dose given at 18 months are known to decline by 5-6 years of age to unprotective levels. Hence it is imperative that the second booster of DPT be given at 5-6 years of age. The recommendation of omitting the 2nd booster probably emerged as the health authorities wanted to concentrate on infants under 1 to 2 years of age under UIP This however has no scientific basis.

Q.49. As per Government instructions only DT is to be given after the age of 2 years. What is your opinion? Should children beyond the age of 2 years not be protected against pertussis ?

This instruction is without any scientific basis. There is no reason not to give DPT vaccine after 2 years. An unvaccinated child remains susceptible throughout life. DPT can be safely given upto 6-7 years of age.

Q.50. A 15 months old child has got injured. The child has received primary series at the right time. What should be done ?

A booster dose of DPT should be given if there is a lapse of 6 months or more, since the last primary dose, besides antiseptic care of the wound.

Q.51. What is Td which is recommended to be given at the age of 10 years ? Is this available ? If not, how do you prepare Td vaccine ?

AKD: Td contains the usual strength of tetanus toxoid (i.e. 10 Lf per dose) but a smaller component of Diphtheria toxoid (4 Lf instead of usual 25 Lf/dose). This is not available in India. In my opinion it should not be prepared by mixing Tetanus toxoid (0.8 ml) and DT (o.2ml) as has been suggested by some.

LK: I do not know of any office procedure by which Td can be prepared.

There does not seem to be any harm in mixing DT and TT in the right proportion to obtain Td, provided the mixing is done just prior to injection.

No child above the age of 7 years should receive either DPT or DT which contain 25 Lf of Diphtheria toxoid, as it causes severe reactions. All these children should be given Td vaccine. In fact some authorities recommend giving Td instead of TT even after injuries to simultaneously boost immunity against both diphtheria and tetanus.

Q.52. Many doctors give a dose of TT after every trivial injury. Is this justified ?

No. It will be determined by the immune status of the individual i.e. whether the child has received tetanus toxoid as DPT, DT or TT and in how many doses. The accompanying table gives the guidelines for rational use of TT and TIG.

Table 1

Guidelines for the use of TT and TIG

TYPE OF WOUND	CLEAN WOUND		OTHER WOUNDS	
Vaccination Status	TT.	TIG	TT	TIG
Unknown or <3 Doses	Yes	No	Yes	Yes
3 or more doses	No	No	No*	No

*Yes if the last dose has been given more than 5 yrs ago.

Tetanus toxoid is a strong immunogenic agent and immunity once achieved, lasts for 5-10 years and hence routine boosters are not required earlier than 10 years. However in cases of deep wounds (e.g burns, trauma) the levels of antitoxin may be inadequate even 5 yrs after the last dose of TT. In such cases a booster may be given if the gap has been 5 or more years.
See also comments (regarding Td) after Q. 49.

Q.53. Is there any hazard of giving unnecessary doses of TT ?

Yes, repeated doses of tetanus toxoid administration may lead to adverse side reactions and theoritically decreased immunity.

Q.54. A 5 year old unvaccinated child has been brought with a contaminated accidental wound. What should be done ?

One dose of DPT to be given immediately and repeated 6-8 wks later followed by booster 6 months later. In addition, tetanus immunoglobulin (TIG) should also be administered at the time of injury in the dose of 250 units I.M.

Q.55. A 6 year old fully vaccinated child has been brought with a contaminated accidental wound. What should be done ?

The wound should be cleaned and dressed aseptically. TT or TIG are not required. Antibiotics may be given as required.

Q.56. Should tetanus immunoglobulin be given to all cases of contaminated wound irrespective of vaccination status ?

No, see Table 1.

Q.57. A 6 months old unvaccinated child is to undergo emergency surgery. Does the child need DPT or tetanus immunoglobulin for protection against tetanus ?

There is no role of giving DPT or DT immediately before an emergency surgery to an unvaccinated child as a minimum of 2 weeks time is required to produce antibodies for protection against the disease. If asepsis cannot be ensured then TIG may be given.

Q.58. Does TIG interfere in development of immunity against tetanus if given concurrently with tetanus toxoid ?

No, but it should be given at separate sites and in two separate syringes.

Q.59. A neonate has been successfully treated for tetanus neonatorum. Should this child also be given DPT series ?

Yes, because tetanus infection does not lead to development of immunity against future infection.

Q.60. Should DPT be avoided in febrile situations or coryza ?

No, mild febrile conditions and common cold are not a contraindication to administering DPT.

It should not be administered at the onset of a coryzal or febrile illness. Running nose is mostly allergic in nature and is not a contraindication to DPT. Mild diarrheal illness is also not a contraindication to DPT.

Q.61. Can DPT be given to a child who has received immunoglobulin in the last 6-8 weeks ?

Yes, it can be given. Only live vaccine administration is to be avoided once immunoglobulin is administered within 8 weeks.

Q.62. Can DPT be given to a child who has suffered from measles 3 weeks back ?

Yes, it can be administered even within 3 weeks of measles as only CMI is decreased after measles while humoral immune response is required following DPT.

Q.63. Can DPT be given to a child receiving long term steroids ?

DPT can be safely given to a child receiving steroids. Only live vaccine are contraindicated in children receiving steroid therapy.

Q.64. Does DPT primary series need to be given to a child who has recovered from diphtheria ?

Yes, as no immunity is induced even after an attack of diphtheria.

Q.65. If DPT is given accidentally to sick child then what problems are anticipated ?

If DPT is given accidentally to a very sick child, it will not be possible to distinguish whether the adverse reactions are due to the original sickness or due to DPT injections.

Some studies in South Africa have shown that there was no increase in adverse reactions even when DPT was given to children at the time of admission to hospital with different illnesses. Nevertheless giving DPT injection during active illness cannot be recommended.

Q.66. A 2 years old child has reported for primary series of DPT. I want to complete the course as early as possible. Can I give DPT injections at weekly interval? Or space the DPT injections at monthly interval and give measles or B C G in between the two doses of DPT ?

For adequate immunological response, 4 weeks is the minimum interval required between two doses of DPT.

Thus weekly doses are not advisable and will not be useful. If DPT is being given at monthly interval then BCG and Measles can be given with the first and third dose of DPT respectively but not in between the two doses of DPT. Administration of two different vaccines if not done on the same day, should not be done at less than 4 weekly interval as otherwise the immunological response to both the vaccines is adversely affected.

Q.67. It has been claimed that only two doses of quadruple vaccine (DPT & killed polio) are required in primary series while if DPT is given alone, three doses are required, why so?

Two doses of quadruple vaccine (DPTP) has been found to give adequate seroconversion if given at 2 and 6 months of age, but no country still advocates the use of two doses of DPTP in their national schedule. Even 2 doses of DPT given at these ages (2 and 6 months) would produce similar immunity. This is not recommended because of the need to complete the schedule as early as possible. The package insert with DPTP still advocates 3 doses at 2, 4 and 6 months of age. Quadruple vaccine is scheduled to be manufactured in India by April, 1992, but the import of this vaccine is not yet allowed in our country.

Q.68. It is said that even after two doses of DPT, adequate protection is achieved against diphtheria and tetanus though not against pertussis. so, if for some reasons a child has to be given DT early then why do we still give three doses of DT ?

Two doses of DT are enough to produce adequate immunity, but in view of the fact that three doses of polio are to be given any way, therefore probably 3 doses of DT are being recommended. Two doses of DT, one each with first and third dose of polio can be given for best response.

Q.69. Immunologists recommend 6-8 weeks as the ideal interval between primary doses of DPT, however the national schedule recommends 4 weeks interval. Kindly clarify.

6 to 8 weeks interval is the ideal interval to produce best immunological response. But in a country like India, Where it is proposed to immunize children as early as possible in life and to have minimum drop out rates, a 4 weeks schedule is being practised. In clinic practice, if one is very sure of his patients,8 weeks schedule can be followed.

Recently immunisation Advisory committee of IAP. has recommended 6-8 weeks interval between successive doses even at national level.

Q.70. Some studies have shown that better seroconversion can be provided with two doses of DPT, if they are spaced at 4 to 6 months interval. Thus, in U.K. only tow primary doses of DPT are given at 2 and 6 months of age. Why do we recommend 3 doses at monthly intervals?

Yes. It is true that adequate seroconversion can be seen with two doses at 4-6 months interval, but the same is not true if the two doses are given at 4 weeks interval. The need to complete the schedule early has compelled us to follow a 3 dose schedule at 6, 10 and 14 weeks, to ensure that complete protection is provided before 4-5 months of age.

Q.71. DPT is available in clear as well as darkly stained ampoules, Why so? Which is better? Does DPT also require protection from light like BCG ?

AKD: The container of DPT vaccine should be clear to observe for any contamination. It is not light sensitive.

LK: Yes, all vaccines should be protected against harsh light.

DPT is not light sensitive. The manufacturers have informed us that they have had to occasionally use coloured ampoules, as clear ampoules were in short supply. It is not clear though, why they still give the instruction of keeping these ampoules in dark.

Q.72. It is always the pertussis fraction which is blamed for reactions. What is there in the pertussis fraction which creates all the problems ?

Presently available pertussis vaccine is a whole cell vaccine which contains many antigenic components which are both toxigenic and immunogenic. This vaccine contains lymphocyte promoting factor (LPF) and filamentous haemagglutination antigen (FHA) which are responsible for reactions. LPF is responsible for neurological disease and FHA is responsible for local reactions.

Q.73. Is there any preparation of DPT likely to be available in near future which will have much less side effects. While retaining its efficacy?

Presently available pertussis vaccine is a whole cell vaccine. It contains many reactogenic substances which are not necessarily immunogenic. Efforts are on to separate those components of pertussis bacill which are immunogenic but not reactogenic. Vaccines made from FHA(filamentous hemaglutination antigen) and/or L.P.F. (Lymphocyte promoting factor) have been tried and found to be successful without producing side effects. These are called acelluar vaccines and are being currently used in Japan, but are not yet available for general use. Acellular vaccines however cannot be used below 2 years of age.

High potency whole cell vaccine which is presently available has proved to be highly efficacious in decreasing the mortality and in controlling the incidence of disease in almost all the countries. None of the acellular vaccine available till now has proven to be as effective as the whole cell vaccine, as shown in trial (1989) conducted in Sweden.

Also it seems that the earlier concern regarding the high incidence of side effects with whole cell vaccine was rather misplaced as recent studies show that the incidence of true reactions attributable to whole cell vaccine is not that high as believed previously. Limited experience with acellular vaccines demonstrate that it has low incidence of side effects when given after 2 years of age, when even whole cell pertussis vaccine has low incidence. In any case pertussis vaccine is required in early infancy where acellular vaccine has not been tried.

Q.74. Can DPT and typhoid be administered at the same sitting at different sites?

DT & Typhod vaccine can be administered at the same sitting at different sites, but not DPT & Typhoid as both of these vaccines are liable to produce febrile reactions.

Bibliography

1. Ad hoc group for the study of pertussis vaccines: Placebo-controlled trial of two acellular pertussis vaccines in Sweden: Protective efficacy and adverse events. Lancet 1:955-960, 1988.
2. American Academy of Pediatrics. Report of the Committee on Infections Desease. Pediatric 1987.
3. Anoyna T, Yuji M, Gondo T, Iwate J. Iwate J. Type specific efficacy of accellular pertussis vaccine. Am J. Dis child 1988, 142: 40-42.
4. Baraff LJ, Leake RD, Borstyn DG et al. Immunologic response to early and routine immunization in infants. Pediatrics 1984, 73: 37-42.
5. Blennow M, Granstrom M, Jaatmaa E, et al: Primary immunization of infants with an acellular pertussis vaccine in a

double blind randemized clinical trial. Pediatrics 1988, 82: 293-299.

6. D.P.T. Guidelines for vaccine prophylaxis and other preventive measures: Recommendation of the Immunization practices Advisory Committee. Anals Int Medicine 1985, 103 : 869-965.
7. Edwards KM, Bradely RB, Decker MD, et al: Evaluation of a new highly purified pertussis vaccine in infants and children. J. Infect Dis 1989, 160: 832-837.
8. Edwards KM and Karzon DT. Pertussis vaccine. Ped Clin North Am. 1990, 37: 549–561.
9. Edwards KM, Lawrence E, Wright PF; Diptheria, tetanus, and pertussis vaccine. A comparison of the immune response and adverse reactions to conventional and acellular pertusis components. Am J Dis Child 140: 867-871, 1986.
10. Larry et al. comparision of DPT manufactured by different pharmaceuticals. Pediatrics 1984, 73: 31-36.
11. Ligham S, Miller C, Pateman J et al. Immunization of preterm infants. Br. Med J. 1986; 292, 1183-35.
12. Linnemann CC et al. Use of pertussis vaccine in an epidemic involving hospital staff. Lancet 1975, 2: 540-543.
13. Marwhich C. Pertussis vaccines trials and tribulations. JAMA 1988, 259: 2057-59.
14. Muller AS et al. Epidemiology and control of pertussis. Tropical Doctor 1987, 17: 182-190.
15. M. Ponteeorvo. DPT in Vaccine sera and immunoglobulin. A practical handbook. Pediatric 1987.
16. Nicoll A et al. Decision making in immunization. BMJ 1988, 297.: 405.
17. Noble GR, Bernier RH, Esber EC, et al; Acellular and whole cell pertussis vaccine in Japan. Report of a visit by US scientists. JAMA 257: 1351,–1356, 1987.
18. Olin P: Comparing the efficacy of pertussis vaccines (letter). Lancet 1989, 1: 95-96.
19. Orenstein WA et al, Diphtheria and tetanus toxoid and pertussis vaccine combined. In : Recent advances in Immunization. A Bibliographic review PAHO Scientific publication. No. 451: 1983, 30-51.
20. Pichichere ME, Badgett JT, Rodgers GC Jr. et al: Acellular pertussis vaccine immunogenicity and safety of an acellular pertussis vs. a whole cell pertussis vaccine combined with diptheria and tetanus toxoids as a booster in 18-24 month old children, Pediatr Infect Dis J 1987, 6: 352-363.

21. Report of the task force on pertussis immunization. Pediatrics (suppl) 1988, 81: 952-984.

22. Roper J, Daya S. Uptake of immunization in low birth weight infants. Am J Dis Child 1986: 63: 518-521.

23. Sharma BK and Chowdhury P: Diphtheria, Pertussis and Tetanus in Immunization Practices In Children. Edited by Dutta A, Mittal SK and Agarwal V. Published by I.A.P. Delhi Branch 1988 pp 11-26.

24. WHO Exp Committee on biological standardization. Tech. Report Series. 638, 1979.

25. Wilkins Jet al. Agglutinin response to pertussis vaccine: Effect of dosage and interval. J. Pediatrics 1971, 79: 197-202.

Killed (or Inactivated) Polio Vaccine (Enhanced potency)

1. **Contents:** Type I 40D, Type II 8D, Type III 32D.
2. **Ideal age of initiating primary vaccination:** 8 wks.
3. **Schedule of primary vaccination:** 3 doses at 6-8 wks interval.
4. **Boosters:** Two, at 1.5 years and 4-5 years.
5. **When recommended:** Routinely & specially in immunocompromised hosts.
6. **Dose** : 0.5ml.
7. **Route of administration:** Intramuscular.
8. **Site of administration:** Anterolateral aspect of thigh.
9. **Preparation of site of administration:** With spirit.
10. **Instructions to the mother after vaccination;** None
11. **Protection/efficacy** : 90-100%.
12. **Contra indications:** None.
13. **Side effects:** Occasional febrile reaction.
14. **Complications:** None reported.
15. **Storage at different levels and at doctor's clinic:**
    a) **When the vaccine is not use:** in lower most compartment of fridge (avoid freezing)
    b) **During immunization session:** Can be kept at room temperature.
    c) **In case of electricity failure:** Keep in cool box.

ORAL POLIO VACCINE (OPV)

1. **Contents:** Sabin attenuated polio virus strain concentration per dose of Type 1: 10^6 TCID50', Type 2 10^5 TCID 50; Type 3: $10^{5.5}$ TCID50
2. **Ideal age of initiating primary vaccination:** 6 weeks (an additional dose recommended at birth by W.H.O.)
3. **Schedule of primary vaccination:** 3 doses at 4 to 8 weeks interval (an optional dose of OPV along with measles vaccination recommended by W.H.O.)
4. **Boosters:** Two, at 1.5 years and between 4-5 years.
5. **When recommended:** Routinely & in epidemic situation.
6. **Dose :** 2 drops.
7. **Route of administration**: Oral.
8. **Site of administration**: Not applicable.
9. **Preparation of site of administration:** Not applicable.
10. **Instructions to the mother after vaccination:** None
11. **Protection/efficacy** : 70-80%.
12. **Contra - indications**: Immunocompromised host or household member.
13. **Side effects**: None.
14. **Complications**: Vaccine induced poliomylites (one in 3 million vaccine)
15. **Storage at different levels and at doctor's clinic:**
    a) **When the vaccine is not use:** Uppermost compartment (2°-4°C) of fridge.
    b) **During immunization session:** On ice.
    c) **In case of electricity failure:** Keep in ice box.

POLIO VACCINE 5

Dr. Jacob John (JJ) & Dr. Meharban Singh (MBS)

Q.1. Schedule of Polio vaccination is most confusing. There is a lot of controversy regarding 3 versus 5 primary doses of polio. What do you recommend ? How many doses would you like your own son or grandson to receive ?

JJ: There is a controversy about the number of doses of OPV, only because people do not understand the principle. If you have only 100 doses, you could give 1 dose to 100 children, 2 doses to 50 children, 3 doses to 33 children. the maximum benefit will be if we gave 1 dose each to 100 children. If enough OPV was available the maximum benefit will be obtained if we give 5 doses to all children, net preference is 4 doses and so forth.

When the Government is giving free vaccine, they have limited it to 3 doses per child. When parents can afford to buy vaccine, they should be advised to give at least 5 doses, preferably 5 for primary and 2 more later.

MBS : In tropical countries, three doses of OPV are inadequate for protection due to interference by enteroviruses and unsatisfactory cold chain management. Unlike USA, three doses of OPV are not sufficient to obtain seroconversion in 100% of infants in India. The Global Advisory Group of WHO has also recommended 4 doses of OPV for primary immunisation in tropical countries with high incidence of acute poliomyelitis. I would like to recommend five doses of OPV (including one dose at birth) for primary immunisation to my son and grandson.

Q.2. Recently WHO has recommended an additional dose of OPV at birth. What is the rationale for this ?

JJ: OPV is effective when given in the neonatal age and thereafter, just like BCG. It is often the first contact period between a health worker and the baby and hence the recommendation for nenoatal OPV.

MBS: Like smallpox vaccination, several studies have shown that transplacental transfer of maternal antibodies against poliomyelitis does not interfere with the take response against OPV. It is true that administration of OPV at birth provides only partial immunity, nevertheless it is useful because of logistic ease of administration. It does reduce the incidence of poliomyelitis during early phase of life in endemic areas and it primes the immune system to respond better to 2nd and subsequent dosages.

OPV at "birth" is most effective when given after 3 days of birth. High content of immunoglobulin in colostrum probably interferes with the uptake of O.P.V. given earlier than that. Studies show that 50% new borns will seroconvert with one dose of OPV.

Q.3. Can preterm children also be given OPV at birth ?

JJ: In the absence of data, I must say yes.

MBS: There is no risk of acquiring poliomyelitis among preterm babies during their nursery stay. The first dose of OPV can be administered to a preterm baby after his discharge from the nursery. There is a need to assess the immunological response of preterm babies to various vaccines which are usually given on the basis of postnatal age rather than conceptional age.

As far as immunological apparatus is concerned, the preterms should be quite capable of reacting to OPV like normal newborns. The preterms should be immunized as per their chronological age like any other new born. But babies still in nursery should not be given OPV as it can then spread to other suscetible hospitalised individuals and can even cause paralytic poliomyelitis in them.

Q.4. In China seven primary doses of OPV are given. Why do they have such a schedule ? What is the basis of this schedule ?

JJ: The Chinese have taken polio control seriously, hence they give 7 doses.

MBS: It is true that seven primary doses of OPV are administered in China, Russia and Malayasia to ensure effective seroconversion for reduction of poliomyelitis. the larger number of doses for primary vaccination are given to safeguard against the possibility of break down in the cold chain system and interference by other enteroviruses.

Better seroconversion rates are obtained with increasing number of trivalent OPV doses. Seven doses would ensure about 95% seroconversion but cannot be recommended because it is neither logistically feasible, nor cost effective.

Q.5. Vaccine containing live viruses or live bacteria are administered in a single dose. Oral Polio is an exception where so many doses have to be given. Why ?

JJ: Because OPV is given by mouth; each time the vaccine is fed; the baby may not respond to it.

MBS: Unlike smallpox vaccination where single dose provides life long immunity, it is true that OPV needs to be administered in multiple doses to achieve satisfactory seroconversion. The sero conversion following three primary doses of OPV ranges between 40% to 75% while following five to six primary doses of OPV it is around 82-96% and 87-100% respectively. The poor seroconversion is related to poor antigenic capabilities of

OPV, thermal lability of vaccine and unsatisfactory maintenance of cold chain and interference by enteroviruses in tropical countries.

Apart from above mentioned factors, a major factor in poor seroconversion with OPV is that it contains 3 serotypes, each one of which is separately antigenic. At one time, one of the serotypes gains a foot hold in the intestinal mucosa and continues to replicate there for next 6-8 wks. This does not allow effective replication of other serotypes, which can then occur only during subsequent doses. Far better seroconversion (85-90%) rates are obtained even with one dose of a monovalent OPV. (See also comment on Q. 6).

Q.6. In the national policy on immunization, it had been mentioned that OPV should be given at an interval of 4 weeks. The American Academy of Pediatrics and Immunization Practices Advisory Committee, US Public Health Service clearly state that "an interval of at least 2 months between the doses of OPV is required because of intestinal carriage of vaccine interference". Kindly clarify this confusion.

JJ: In the vast majority of babies vaccine viruses disappear within 4 weeks. Hence the minimum gap recommended is 4 weeks.

MBS: The interval between primary doses of OPV should not be less than 4 weeks to ensure adequate seroconversion. It is true that increased intervals (6 to 8 weeks) are equally satisfactory but it is desirable that interval between the primary doses of OPV should be restricted to 4 weeks so that the schedule can be completed and the child is protected at an early age considering that the disease is endemic in our country.

It is true that vaccine virus may persist upto 6 weeks in the intestinal mucosa and therefore a second dose of OPV given after 8 weeks of the primary dose is far more effective then given at 4 weeks interval. U.S.A. regularly gives 3 doses at 8 weeks interval. Even two studies done in India which employed a 6 or 8 weeks interval between consecutive doses, also obtained as good a seroconversion rates with 2 or 3 doses, as have been obtained later by 5 doses given at 4 weeks interval. This 4 weeks interval is probably an important factor responsible for poor seroconversion observed in most of the studies after 3 doses. However, the imperative need to complete the schedule as early as possible and to minimise the drop outs, a period of 4 weeks has been practised in this country. This is also effective but less than that of 6-8 weeks. Recently Immunization advisory committee of I.A.P. has suggested a dose schedule at 6-8 weeks interval for OPV even in India. It would probably be possible to achieve adequate seroconversion even with 3 doses given at 8 weeks interval even in our country. Thus if we wish to follow a 4 week interval we must give 5 doses, but if we can practice 8 weeks interval probably 3 doses would suffice.

Q.7. Interference with other enteroviruses is believed to be one of the major reasons of decreased efficacy of polio vaccine in tropical countries like India. Should we then avoid giving polio vaccine in summer ? Should we give more doses in summer or should we try killed vaccine in summer?

JJ: There is no need to follow seasonal immunization.

MBS: The babies are being born round the year and it would be dangerous to leave them unimmunised during summer months due to endemic nature of poliomyelitis in India. The administration of five primary doses of OPV, irrespective of the seasons, shall ensure adequate protection to majority of children. Administration of IPV during summer is desirable and useful but there are logistic difficulties.

It is impractical to use two different schedules (or different vaccines) for summers and winters.

Q.8. What is the efficacy of 3 doses of oral polio vaccine?

JJ: Efficacy varies according to geographic regions; maximum 89% (temperate regions) minimum about 75% (tropical regions).

MBS: As already emphasized vide supra, three primary doses of OPV (4 weeks interval) are inadequate for satisfactory sero conversion and protection of vulnerable population.

Three doses given at 8 weeks interval provide much high seroconversion rates (85%-95%) even in tropical regions.

Q.9. Many studies indicate that seroconversion (development of immunity) is better with two IM doses of killed vaccine than the five doses of OPV. However, we continue to use oral polio only. why?

JJ: Because of (a) national policy of OPV (b) lack of free availability of IPV and (c) high cost of IPV.

MBS: There is a marginal superiority of IPV as compared to OPV for seroconversion especially pertaining to antibody response against polio type 3. Several studies from France have demonstrated identical efficacy of OPV and IPV to the tune of seroconversion rates of 98-100% if potency of OPV is ensured by optimal cold chain management. In our country five primary doses of OPV are recommended because it is cheap, easy to administer, provides gut immunity and is acceptable to the community. The major problem is the need for maintenance of strict cold chain and there is certainly a need to evolve a relatively heat resistant OPV.

Previously the IPV which was available had low antigenic content and did not give rise to as good seroconversion rates as OPV. That is why OPV was preferred in our country. Recently an imporved version of IPV (with 40D,

8 D and 32 D content of Type I, II & III polio serotypes respectively) has become available. This enhanced potency IPV (IPV-Ep) is definitely more immunogenic and consistently provides good seroconversion rates, with 3 doses at 2, 4 & 6 months or with 2 doses at 2 & 6 months of age. the vaccine is very costly compared to OPV and besides, being a killed parenteral vaccine, it does not provide any gut immunity and hardly any 'herd effect'. It may not be helpful in curbing the circulation of wild virus in the community which is essential for ultimate eradication of the disease. Thus while IPV may be good for individual protection, its role as a "community vaccine" is doubtful. Nevertheless the Government of India, Ministry of Biotechnology has decided to set up a plant for manufacturing IPV. It will start producing IPV very soon. It can also be combined with DPT and be made available as quadruple vaccine (DPTP) This quadruple vaccine will also be manufactured in the country. There is a great need to conduct studies for assesing the feasibility, efficacy and cost effectiveness of both IPV & DPTP (quadruple vaccine) in our own country so that when these vaccines become available, they can be utilized optimally.

Heat resistant OPV is an Utopia and till that is achieved, IPV may be a better alternative, for individual protection.

Q.10. It is said that development of local gut immunity is important in preventing an attack of poliomyelitis. When we use only killed vaccine, what happens to the gut immunity ?

JJ: Gut immunity is less important than systemic immunity. IPV induces higher systemic and lower gut immunity.

MBS : It is logical to assume that there is no development of gut immunity following IPV but no epidemiological data is available to confirm this belief.

The presence of gut immunity is important, it helps to prevent the wild virus from getting a foot hold in the

intestinal mucosa. Nevertheless the systemic immunity is even more important in preventing the disease, as it prevents the spread of virus to the target organs (viz the anterior horn cells). If adequate systemic immunity is there, even the virus may not be able to get a foot hold in the intestines as there is an extermely good blood supply there also, and in any case the disease is extermely unlikely.
Recently it has been shown that with IPV-Ep, some gut immunity also develops.

Q.11. Has the incidence of poliomyelitis decreased in the last 10 years after EPI ?

JJ: Probably not.

MBS: We do not have any authentic data regarding the incidence of poliomyelitis in India. Most hospitals and survey data tend to show that the incidence of poliomyelitis has not significantly decreased over the past 10 years. It is estimated that the incidence of poliomyelitis in India ranges between 2 to 3 lacs every year which is equivalent to 500-700 new cases every day or one child is affected every 2 minutes in the country. The poor impact of EPI programme on the incidence of poliomyelitis, may be due to inadequate coverage, increasing population, better reporting system and poor protection due to poorly stored, impotent polio vaccine.

Recent data (1989-1990) from sentinel centres at Madras, Bombay and even at Delhi, show that there is some decline in the incidence of poliomylitis in our country. Whether this represents a periodic reduction in incidence (following high incidence year of 1987-1988) or an impact of better polio vaccine coverage (and hence sustainable), remains to be seen. In any case even today (Jan, 1991) our vaccine coverage remains far from satisfactory and we do not seem to be anywhere near the UIP goal of 85% coverage of infants all over the country. Not only must we achieve this goal, but also we should be able to sustain it for minimum 3-5 years before we can expect substantial reduction in the incidence.

Q.12. Why do we get polio cases even after complete schedule of polio vaccination ? Is it that the vaccine is not fully effective ?

JJ: Such cases are examples of "vaccine failure". If vaccine efficacy is less than 100% then vaccine failure cases would occur.

MBS: Poliomyelitis may occur in vaccinated children either due to poor seroconversion with even potent vaccines or more commonly due to the use of impotent vaccine.

About 10-12% cases of polio reported at Kalawati Saran Children hospital, New Delhi, occur among completely immunised children. Similary in cities like Madras where more than 90% population is covered with O.P.V., 30% of all case of polio admitted to Institute of Child Health, occur among immunized children. Statiscally even these figures suggest a 85% efficacy of O.P.V. Also clinical and epidemiological data from Haffkine Institute, Bombay indicates that three dose of OPV have a 85% efficacy in clinical situations. Although this interpretation may be doubted, but the fact remains that even 3 doses, as being practised now, have considerable clinical efficacy. Efficacy can be increased by either giving 5 doses or by spacing 3 primary doses at 8 weeks interval.

Most cases, of vaccine failure occur due to Type 2 polio virus and less commonly due to Type 3. Rarely these are due to Type 1.

It must be remembered that despite occassional vaccine failure, majority of cases in our country still occur among unimmunised individuals.

Q.13. Is the severity of poliomyelitis in post vaccination cases less than in unvaccinated case ?

JJ: Probably yes, but there is no data to support it.

MBS: There is no significant difference regarding the age of onset, clinical spectrum and severity of poliomyelitis among vaccinated and unvaccinated children, However, the recovery of paralysis is faster and better among vaccinated children.

Q.14. What is the incidence of polio vaccine induced poliomyelitis ?

The overall incidence of post vaccinial poliomyelitis following OPV in children is around one in three million and in adults it is around one in two million vaccinees.

Q.15. Polio vaccine (OPV), given to adults can lead to paralytic polio. Is there any substance in this statement?

It is true that OPV given to a seronegative (susceptible) adults may be followed by paralytic poliomyelitis due to vaccinial virus. In developed countries, OPV whether given to children or adults, does pose a significant risk of vaccine related poliomyelitis and there is an increasing trend and rethinking towards the use of inactiviated polio vaccine.

Vaccine induced poliomyelitis has become one of the major concerns today in the developed countries where the incidence of wild virus polio is almost negligible. It has been estimated that vaccine induced poliomyletits occurs in I case after 5,20,000 first dose of OPV. Although only 10% cases out of these, occur in immunocompromised hosts, but the incidence in them is increased about 10,000 times compared to that in normal individuals Even immunocompromised contacts of the vaccinees are at increased danger of developing vaccine induced poliomyelitis. The concern has greatly increased in recent times because of increasing incidence of AIDS is these countries.

Because of these concerns, there is a considerable rethinking in USA where it has been suggested that IPV be given to immunocompromised individuals and recently FDA of USA has sanctioned the use of IPV Ep for general vaccination. It has also been suggested that a combined schedule of IPV (one dose) followed by two doses of OPV be practised to prevent problem of vaccine induced poliomyelitis, while producing complete and long lasting immunity.

In any case vaccine induced paralysis is only a theoritical problem in our country as almost all of our paralytic polio is still due to wild polio virus.

Q.16. Is there any chance that live oral attenuated polio vaccine virus can become virulent by repeated passages through unvaccinated (susceptible) infants and children and cause clinical polio ?

It is true that attenuated polio virus contained in OPV may become virulent by repeated passages through unvaccinated infants and children assuming the characteristics of wild virus thus leading to paralytic attacks.

Serotype 3 of vaccins virus is the one which reverts most easily from its attenuated strain to a virulent strain and hence is most likly to cause vaccine induced poliomyelits. Research is currently going on to improve this companent of O.P.V.

Q.17. It has been said that vaccine induced paralytic poliomyelitits can occur even upto 6 months after administration of OPV. Thus how can we distinguish these (vaccine induced) cases from those due to vaccine failure ?

These cases cannot be distinguished clinically. Only way to distinguish them is by virological methods. If a child develops paralytic polio and his stool grows polio vaccine virus, then the case may be considred to be due to vaccine itself. (Strictly speaking even this evidence is not adequate as the paralysis may be due to other enteroviruses also). On the other hand if the stool grows one of the wild polio virus strains (usually type II or III) then this is a case of vaccine failure.

Q.18. W.H.O. has recommended giving OPV in diarrhea but not counting it. What does it mean ?

It is desirable that every contact of the child with heath personnel should be exploited for administration of vaccines. There is no harm to administer OPV in children with mild to moderate diarrhea but since the 'take' response is questionable, it is recommended that such doses should not be counted and child should be administered an additional dose of OPV when he has recovered from diarrhea.

Q.19. Accidentally I have given 7-8 drops of oral polio vaccine instead of 2 drops to an infant. What commplications are anticipated ?

There is no risk with administration of a higher dose of OPV but one should use only the recommended dose.

Clinical experience tells that mild diarrhea may occur in these cases.

Q.20. I got a case who had been injected OPV by mistake. The parents wanted to know what reactions may occur. Can you tell us the consequences of such a situation ?

Accidental injection of OPV has been reported not only from India but from other countries including France and Chekoslavakia also. There is no serious risk following intra muscular injection of OPV except theoretical risk of necrosis of muscle due to magnesium chloride content of the vaccine. There is no risk of development of poliomyelitis. The immune response is practically nil following parenteral administration of OPV and vaccination should be continued by giving adequate OPV doses per oral.

Q.21. Fifth dose of OPV is being recommended with measles vaccination. As both these vaccines are live virus vaccines, should these vaccines be given concurrently ?

The OPV can be concurrently administered with measles vaccine without any interference or side effects.

Q.22. Fifth dose of polio (primary series) according to WHO schedule is 'Optional'. Please clarify how to exercise this option ?

JJ: Where vaccine failures are common after 3 or 4 doses, 5 doses are recommended.

MBS: There is a progressive increase in sero positivity following additional doses of OPV. It is preferable to give five primary doses of OPV (including one dose given at or soon after birth along with BCG). The fifth dose can be given along with measles vaccine.

When WHO says the 5th dose is optional, it means it is optional for different member countries, whether to incorporate it in their national immunization programmes or not. If the epidemiological data of a particular country shows that even after giving 4 doses (at birth, 6, 10 & 14 weeks) the response is inadequate, then it may also incorporate the 5th dose. Recommendations of using it simultaneously with measles is mainly for logistic reasons (number of visits). The immunisation advisory committee of I.A.P. has in any case recommended giving the 5th dose of OPV with measles vaccine at 8 months of age.

Q.23. One dose of OPV was given at birth. The infant has reported at the age of 6 months. Should the dose of OPV at birth be counted or five more doses of OPV be given to such a child ?

The dose of OPV already given should be counted irrespective of the lapsed interval.

Q.24. Should we not give six primary doses (one at birth and five primary doses) of OPV to precious children ?

Every child is precious and we should give five primary doses of OPV (including one dose given at or soon after birth).

Q.25. What should be the interval between the last primary dose of polio vaccine and the 1st booster dose ?

The booster dose should be given after 6 months to one year, of the last primary dose of OPV.

Q.26. How many booster doses of OPV do you recommend ?

Two booster doses of OPV should be given, one at one and half years and second around 4-5 yrs of age (school entry).

Once a seroconversion has been achieved with primary doses of OPV there is no further need of boosters with OPV, because oral polio vaccine being a live attenuated virus, it continues to be replicated in the intestine. But as in our country, the serocoversion with 3 or even 5 primary doses cannot be considered to be 100%, it may still be desirable to give at least one booster (infact reinforcing dose) at 1.5 year of age. Value of any further dose, is highly debatable particularly in view of the fact that almost 100% children in our country would have any way developed natural immunity by 5 years of age.

On the other hand with IPV, although sereconversion is obtained in 100% following 3 doses, yet no permanent mechanism (like stimulation of memory cells) is set up in the body. Hence these children require boosters at 1.5 years and at 5 years. Manufacturers of IPV-Ep (presently available) claim that you may not require boosters following 3 primary doses of IPV-Ep but this claim has not yet been substantiated in any controlled trial.

Q.27. Some authorities recommend OPV booster every year. What are your comments on this schedule ?

There is no need to give OPV booster every year. Some authorities even recommend boosters of OPV every five years among children and every 10 years among adults, but this is also not required.

Q.28. What is the rationale of omitting the booster dose at 5 years of age which used to be followed earlier in the national schedule ?

There is no rationale of omitting the booster dose of OPV at 5 years of age except due to logistic difficulties and shortage of vaccine. It is recommended that school authorities should enforce that all children are adequately immunized before they are accepted for admission.

In the national schedule, at present, 2nd booster at 4.5 to 5 yrs of age is not recommended. It is mainly because the immunisation programme is mostly concentrating on infants less than 1 year of age and also because most children acquire antibodies in our country by 3-5 years of age and hence probably do not require further doses.

Q.29. In ICDS projects, OPV is recommended till the age of 2 yrs - why ?

JJ: Because the risk of polio is highest under 2 years of age.

MBS: The target population for universal programme of immunisation is limited to infants upto one year of age due to their enhanced vulnerability, logistic convenience and availability of vaccine stock. In ICDS projects since children under the age of 6 years are under surveillance they should get at least two boosters, of polio.

The government argues that children above 2 years have been excluded from National Immunisation

Programme against polio, mainly because majority of children by that age have already acquired antibodies by means of subclinical infections. In fact by 3 years of age, more than 90% of children have protective polio antibodies and may not require any further doses of polio. These arguments are not totally acceptable and in any case when dealing with an individual child, no risk can be taken. It is therefore still recommended that all children upto 5-6 years of age should receive complete protection against poliomyelitis.

Q.30. What should be the schedule of polio vaccination of an unvaccinated 2 years old child who has reported for the first time ?

JJ: Give 3 doses under EPI or 5 doses, if parents will purchase OPV.

MBS: The two year old unvaccinated child should receive 3 doses of OPV at an interval of one month each followed by one booster after one year and second booster after 3 years.

Q.31 Can any combination of killed and oral polio vaccine give better results than either vaccine given alone ?

It is suggested that first dose of IPV should be given followed by subsequent 4 doses of OPV in order to reduce the incidence of vaccine associated paralytic poliomyelitis and to reduce the risk of fecal transmission of polio virus. In Gaza, combination of OPV and IPV has virtually eradicated poliomyelitis.

Q.32. Till what age polio vaccination may be given ? In other words, after what age polio vaccination is not required ?

In developing countries, with very high chances of oro-fecal contamination, due to unsatisfactory sanitory conditions, the administration of polio vaccine is usually unwarranted beyond the age of 5 years.

Q.33. Which vaccines can be given concurrently with OPV and which vaccines can not be given concurrently with OPV ?

Any vaccine can be given concurrently with OPV.

Q.34. Can we hope to eradicate polio with existing programmes ?

JJ: With existing vaccine yes, but with the present strategy, no.

MBS: It is not possible to eradicate poliomyelities with the existing UIP-EPI programme which are aimed at reducing the incidence of poliomyelitis rather than actual eradication.

UIP aims at 85% coverage of under 1 year olds. Almost half the doses of polio vaccine tested at various centres are not found to be potent. Even 3 doses of potent vaccine given to 100% individuals, allows seroconversion only in about 70%. Therefore with 85% coverage and 50% potency one can expect effective protection in only about 30% of children. This obviously is not sufficient to eradicate polio from any community.

Q.35. In recent times, the Government of India has taken number of steps to improve cold chain conditions and thus to improve overall potency of available OPV. What are the results of these steps and do you think we are now in a better position to eradicate polio with continued use of OPV as suggested under UIP?

It is true that a number of steps have been taken under the UIP to improve the cold chain status. Also facilities for potency testing of vaccine have been considerably strengthened. As a result more than 80 to 90% of vaccine samples tested at NICD Delhi in 1989-1990, have been found to be potent. This is an extremely encouraging trend. However we still feel that even with better cold chain facilities, just routine administration of OPV will not eradicate poliomyletts even if we achieve 85% coverage of all infants and sustain it for more than 5 years as envisaged under UIP.

It must be remembered that almost all the countries in the world, which have eradicated polio with the help of OPV, have done so by initialing programme of simultaneous mass immunisation of susceptible polulation at the begining of the progamme and then maintaining high rates of immunisation through routine immunisation services. There is still no country in the world which has eradicated poliomy elitis by using routine OPV immunisation alone, as suggested under EPI or UIP.

Q.36. What is pulse Immunisation (for polio)?

The pulse immunisation programme referes to intermittent polio immunization drive in a community or a region, to vaccinate all susceptible children irrespective of their previous immunisation status. This helps to establish the vaccine virus in the community and to replace the wild virus by the vaccine virus. Cuba, Brazil, Israel etc have successfully eradicated polio by using the pulse method. In our country also, it has been shown in Vellore that the use of cluster or pulse approach can reduce the incidence of poliomyelitis by 90% within three months. Pulse programme, however, should complement the conventional, schedule oriented, EPI programme (For principle of pulse Immunisation, see Chapter on General consideration)

Q.37. Pulse immunisation has almost eradicated poliomyelitis from several countries like Brazil. Why do we not adopt such a policy for our country ?

The major bottleneck against pulse programme in our country is the large number of susceptible children (approximately 100 million) and enormous size of the country. There is a need for political will, monetary sanctions and availability of at least 250 million indigenously manufactured OPV doses per year for annual pulse campaigns alone, in the country.

Mass coverage of children with O.P.V. which ensures eradication of wild polio virus is the most effective and quickest way of eradicating poliomyelitis and lack of resources should not deter us from undertaking this exercise. Similary large size of our country is also not a problem as Brazil is as large as our country (in size). In any case the country has successfully held a large number of general elections ensuring 1 ballot box for each 1000 population, why it can't provide 1 vaccine box for every 500-1000 children once or twice every year is beyond comprehension. This only shows lack of political will.

Q.38. What should be donc to prolect children during polio epidemic ?

all under - 5 year children should be given one dose of OPV (irrespective of their immunisation status). DPT and other intra-muscular injections and surgical operations like tonsillectomy should be withheld during an epidemic and public awareness should be created to prevent orofecal transmission of poliovirus.

Q.39. You have said that tonsillectomy and intramuscular injections should be avoided during polio epidemics Why ?

Intramuscular injections & tonsillectomy during an epidemic of poliomyelitis enhances the risk of paralytic poliomyelitis and its severity. The raw area at the tonsillar bed or inflammation at intramuscular injection site, elicits reflex vascular response in the corresponding segment of the spinal cord leading to migration of poliovirus along the axons to the anterior horn cells.

Q.40. If the water supply is contaminated with Polio vaccine virus, would this not curb the circulation of wild virus in the community and decrease the incidence of polio markedly ?

JJ : No.

MBS: The contamination of water supply with the attenuated poliovirus is an exciting possibility but is assciated with the risk of emergence of wilder strain of poliovirus following its several passages through susceptible individuals with increased risk of vaccine-related poliomyelitis. Moreover, the virus may lose its potency due to increased environmental temperature.

This cannot be recommended.

Q.41. Should polio vaccine be given to those children who have already suffered or are suffering from poliomyelitis ?

There is a need to administer trivalent OPV in attack of acute poliomyelitis to safegurard against the occurence of poliomyelitis due to other serotypes of polio virus.

Q.42. How soon after an attack of poliomyelitis, should OPV be administered ?

OPV should be administered after least 4 to 8 weeks of an attack of acute poliomyelitis.

Q.43. Can administration of polio vaccine in the prodromal and preparalytic stage of poliomyelitis help in preventing an attack of paralytic polio ?

JJ: No.

MBS: OPV may prevent or modify an attack of poliomyelitis if given during the early incubation period but will be ineffective when administered during the prodromal or preparalytic stage of poliomyelitis.

Q.44. A child developed an acute episode of diarrhea 12 hours after ingestion of OPV. Is this a side effect or incidental ? Should this dose be counted or not ?

The occurrence of an episode of diarrhea 12 hours after the ingestion of OPV is merely incidental. There is no need to disregard this dose of OPV because 4 to 6 hours are enough for the virus to be absorbed through lymphatics and to take hold in the intestinal musoa.

Q.45. Is it true that diarrhea can develop after polio vaccination? Which drugs should be prescribed to children who develop diarrhea after polio drops administration ?

JJ: Yes, diarrhea can develop after OPV. Only ORS should be given to such cases.

MBS: Diarrhea is not a known side effect of OPV and the child should be managed as any other case of acute gastroenteritis.

There is no mention in the literature which indicates diarrhea as a side effect of OPV. However one often sees children who have mild diarrhea following OPV administration which usually has no consequence. Any moderate or severe diarrhea following OPV should be taken as an independent episode of gastro enteritis and managed as such.

Q.46. What instruction should be given to the mother after OPV administration ?

The mother does not need any specific instructions following administration of OPV except that she should be reminded to report for subsequent immunization at the proper time.

Q.47. Presently it is recommended that breast feeding can be given just before and soon after OPV administration. Why was it recommended otherwise earlier ? What new data has accumulated to make the present recommendations? Is the polio vaccine being made these days breast milk resistant?

The recent data suggests that breast feeding does not inactivate OPV and the infant can be given breast feeding just before or soon after administration of OPV. Colostrum may interfere with 'take' response of OPV while mature breast milk does not pose any significant interference.

Q.48. Can hot liquids be given soon after OPV administration ?

The mother can give a bottle feed (if child was already top fed), after administration of OPV. Of course she should make sure that the milk is not too hot to produce any scalds.

Q.49. If polio vaccine is regurgitated within one hour of administration, should the dose be repeated ?

It is preferable to repeat the dose of OPV if the previous dose has been regurgitated within one hour of administration.

Q.50. Can polio vaccine (OPV) be given to children on steroid therapy (compromised hosts)?

OPV should not be given in immunocompromised patients and children receiving daily steroid therapy in high doses.

IPV should be given in such cases. OPV should be avoided not only in such individuals, but even in their close contacts.

Q.51. Can polio vaccine be given to a child who has recovered from measles ?

JJ: Yes

MBS: OPV should be administered after one month following an attack of measles.

Q.52. Can polio vaccine be given to a child who has received immunoglobulin a month back ?

The administration of all live vaccines including OPV should be delayed at least 6 weeks following an injection of immunoglobulin.

Q.53. Can polio vaccine be given to a child who is suffering from chicken pox ?

MBS: There is no logic or need to administer OPV to a child who is suffering from chicken pox and vaccine should be postpond for at least one month after the attack.

JJ: Not recommended, except in epidemic situation.

Q.54. Can polio vaccine be given to a child who is on antirabies post-exposure prophylaxis ?

There is no contraindication for administration of OPV to a child receiving antirabies prophylaxis.

Q.55. Can polio vaccine be given to a child with hepatitis ?

As a general rule all vaccines are contraindicated in a child suffering from acute illnesses including hepatitis.

Q.56. Can polio vaccine be given to a child suffering from AIDS or who is in close contact with such a patient.

There is a generalised depression of immunity in patients with AIDS and hence knowing the capacity of OPV to produce paralytic poliomyelitis in immunocompromised hosts (or family contacts) it would be logical not to give OPV to such cases. However no reaction has been observed in a few cases of AIDS who have been accidently given OPV in USA. Nevertheles it is prudent to avoid OPV and instead to give IPV in such cases.

Whenever it is considered urgent to give polio vaccine, and OPV cannot be given bacause of one or the other reasons, (like measles, chicken pox etc.) then IPV can be safely given.

Q.57. What are the contraindications to oral polio vaccination?

The main contraindications to OPV include, acute fabrile illness, severe diarrhea, immunocompromised host and pregnancy. In all these cases, IPV can be given if required.

Q.58. Are all available polio vaccine (OPV) light pink in color ?

Yes all currently available polio vaccines are light pink in colour due to phenol red which is used as a pH indicator.

Q.59. If the color of the vaccine has faded, does it mean that the vaccine has lost its potency ?

JJ: No

MBS: Phenol red gets bleached when exposed to light and faded vaccine is indicative of poorly preserved or possibly impotent vaccine.

Manufacturers of OPV indicate that variation in colour is not indicative of lost potency. It may still be preferable to get potency testing of such vials.

Q.60. Does yellow discoloration of vaccine indicates signs of bacterial contamination? Kindly explain the basis of this phenomenon ?

MBS: The appearance of yellow discoloration along with turbidity is strongly suggestive of contamination of the vacine with bacteria. The metabolism of the bacterial cell lowers the pH of the vaccine, leading to change in the colour and turbidity.

JJ: Acidity causes yellow colour while alkalinity leads to pink colour.

Q.61. What is the failure rate of OPV inspite of maintaining adequate cold chain ?

JJ: Failure rate varies in different regions.

MBS: The poor maintenance of cold chain system (either at manufacturer, central supply, regional supply, transport from health post to the community or at the time of administration etc) is the commonest cause of vaccine failure. The other important reasons for poor protection following vaccination with OPV include poor immunological response on the part of the host due to genetic factors and competitive inhibition by other enteroviruses in the gut.

Epidemiologically, it is difficult to differentiate cases of vaccine failure due to cold chain failure and those due to 'true' vaccine failure. It is to be noted that seroconversion rate with even 3 doses of potent vaccine, is not more than 70% and hence cases of vaccine failure can also be expected.

Q.62. How to preserve polio vaccine (in which compartment of the refrigerator) ?

The OPV should preferably be placed in the top most compartment of refrigerator just below the freezer at a temperature of + 4°C to + 8°C. The vaccine vial not in current use can be kept in the freezer compartment but frequent thawing and freezing is inadvisable. The vaccine should be transported in ice boxes or isothermic boxes by using cold accumulators (cold packs) and ice cubes.

Q.63. How to maintain polio vaccine:

(a) When not in use ?

It should be stored in the deep freze at - 20°C temperature for bulk stock (viability one year) and between + 4°C to + 8°C (viability 3 months) for storage in the hospital/post/clinic. No vaccine should ever be kept in the door of refrigerator.

(b) During immunization session ?

The cold accumulators (cold packs) and water bottles (not for drinking purposes) should be kept in the refrigerator to ensure that temperature is maintained for at least 2-4 hours during electricity failure. In the event of a prolonged breakdown, the vaccine should be transferred isothermic boxes containing plenty of ice. If electrical failure is a perpetual problem, the availability of a generator or refrigerator run by gas/petrol are mandatory.

(d) If the doctor is not having fridge in his clinic ?

All pediatricians/physicians who are dispensing vaccination must acquire a refrigerator their clinics.

Q.64. As per government instructions, once a vial is opened the left over vaccine should be discarded after the immunisation session, while practitioners keep the left over vaccine in the refrigerator for further use. What is your opinion about such a practice ?

There is no harm in keeping the left over vaccine in the refrigerator for further use as long as sterility and cold chain stipulations are strictly maintained. Freezing and thawing should however be avoided.

Q.65. How much ice should be put in a thermos to make sure of polio preservation? how can we know the temperature inside the thermos ?

The vaccine in the thermos flask should be surrounded by ice from below, above and sides. The temperature inside the flask can be determined with the help of a thermometer.

As long as there is enough unmelted ice in the thermos, the temperature inside is probably alright.

Q.66. The vaccine is available as a multiple dose vial in which we have to inject the needle repeatedly. Some companies supply in the form of tube with a dropper. Which is better to use in our practice ? What is your comment on this ?

It is preferable to use OPV vials which are provided with a dropper. The repeated punctures of multiple dose vial with injection needle is fraught with the risk of contamination and bacterial infection.

Q.67. Do you think that polio drops should be made available in single dose vials ?

Single dose vials of OPV may appear convenient for practitioners dispensing small number of doses every day. However, they will be more expensive and would require much greater space for storage in the cold chain system.

Q.68. I always get worried about the potency of polio drops. Can't I get them tested ?

It is feasible to get the potency of OPV checked in a reputed virology laboratory such as National Institute of Communicable Diseases, Delhi and Haffkine Institute, Bombay. The impotent vaccine must be discarded.

The vaccine should be transported under cold chain stipulations when being sent for testing, mentioning the batch number of vaccine. You can expect the report in 3-4 weeks time.

Bibliography

1. Advisory committee on Immunization Practices (ACIP: New Recommended schedule for active immunization of normal infants and children. MMWR 1986, 35: 577.
2. Arya SC; Continuing global polioyelitis morbidity and lacunae of trivalent poliovirus vaccines. Vaccine 1988, 6: 213.

3. Bass JW, Halstead SB, Fisher GW, et al; Oral polio vaccine Effect of booster vaccination one to 14 years after primary series. JAMA 1978, 239: 2252.
4. Bernier RH: Imroved inactivated poliovirus vaccine: An update. Pediatr Infect Dis 1896, 5: 289.
5. Chaudhary DS, Nossik NN, Bindee P et al. Poliomyelitis vaccination of infants : Pre-immunization status and sero conversion. Bull WHO 1973; 48 : 195-98.
6. Cherry JD: Enteroviruses. In Behrman RE, Vaughan VC (eds) z: Nelson Textbook of Pediatrics, ed 13. Philadelphia, WB Saunders Company, 1989, p 689.
7. Committe on Infectious Diseases Active and passive immunization. In 1988 Red Book, ed 21. Elk Grove Village, Illinois, American Academy of Pediatrics, 1988, p 5.
8. Dave, KH: Study of poliomyelitis in Bombay in Sentinal Surveillance, Ed. Basu RN Epidemiology division, National Institute of Communicable diseases, Delhi, 1985, 50-55.
9. De-Xiaing D, Xi-min H, Wan-Jun L, et al; Immunization of neonates with trivalent oral poliomyelitis vaccine (Sabin). Bull WHO 1986, 64: 853.
10. Gaebler JW, Kleiman MB, French MLV, et al: Neurologic complications in oral poliovaccine recipient. J Pediatr 1986,108: 878.
11. Ghosh S, Kumari S, Balaya S. et al. Antibody response to Oral Polio vaccine in infancy. Indian Pediatrics 1970, 7 : 78
12. Halsey N, Galazka A: The efficacy of DTP and oral poliomyelitis immunization schedules initiated from birth to 12 weeks of age. Bull WHO 1985, 63: 1151.
13. Hinman AR, Koplan JP, Urenstein WA, et al: Live or inactivated p olimyelitis vaccine: An analysis of benefits and risks. Am J Public Health 1989, 77: 1.
14. Huovilainen A, Kinnunen L, Ferguson M, et al: Antigenic Variation among 173 strains of type 3 poliovirus isolated in Finland during the 1984 to 1985 outbreak. J. Gen Virol 1988, 69: 1941.
15. Idris MS, Mathur A, sharma P et al. Oral Polio vaccine and factors affecting its effcacy. I J M R 1980, 71:68.
16. John TJ, Devarajan LV, Luther L, et al: Effect of breast feeding on serorespense of infants to oral poliovirus vaccination. Pediatrics 1976, 57: 47.
17. John TJ, P andian R, Gadomski A, et al: Control of poliomyelitis by pulse immunization in vellore, India. Br Med J 1983, 286: 31.

18. John TJ: Poliomyelitis in India — Prospects and problems of control. Rev Infect Dis. 1984: 6 (suppl 2) 438-41.

19. John TJ: Immunization against poliomyelitis—Present concepts and practices. Indian J Pub health 1958; 29: 3, 162-67.

20. John TJ: Immune response of neonates to oral poliomyelitis vaccine, Br. Med J 289: 881, 1984.

21. John TJ. Antibody response of infants in tropics to 5 doses of OPV. BMJ 1976; 811-12.

22. John TJ. Revised immunization schedule of the WHO Expanded programme on Immunization. Ind pediatr 1988, 25: 3-6.

23. Khare S, Dutta M, Lal B, Kumari S. Quality control of cold chain system-Potency testing of OPV vaccine. commun. dis Bull 1988, 5: 9-13.

24. Kim-Farely R, Dave KH, Sokhey J and mandke VB. Poliomyelitis surveillance and vaccin efficancy. Bombay EPI-1988.

25. McBear AM Thom ML Johnson RH. A comparison of the serologic responses to oral and injectable trivallent oral polio vaccine. Rev Infect Dis 1984; 6 : suppl 2 : 552-55.

26. Melnick JL: Polomyelitis vaccines: An appraisal after 25 years. Comp Ther 1980, 5:6.

27. Melnick JL: Live attenuated oral poliovirus vaccine. Rev Infect Dis 1984, 6 (suppl 2) 323.

28. Sabin AB: Vaccination against poliomyelitis in economically under-developed countries. Bull WHO 1980, 58 : 141 - 151.

29. Sabin AB. Vaccine control of poliomelitis in the 80's Yale J Biol Med 1982; 55: 383-89.

30. Sabin AB: Oral poliovirus vaccine: History of its development and use and current challange to eliminate poliomyelitis from the world. J Infect Dis 1985, 151: 420.

31. Salk J: Commentary: Poliomyelitis vaccination-Choosing a wise policy. Pediatr Infect Dis 1987, 6:889.

32. Sen S. Poliomyelitis in Immunization Practices in children. Ed. A Datta SK Mittal and V Agarwal Ind Acad Padiatrics, Delhi 1988.

33. Schoub BD, Johnson S, McAnerny J, et al: Monovalent neonatal polio immunization. A strategy for the developping world. J Infect Dis 157: 836, 1988.

34. Simoes EAF, Padmini B, Stenhoff MD, Jadhav M, John TJ. Antibody response of infants to 2 doses of IPV of enhanced potency. Am J Dis Child 1985; 139: 977-80.

MEASLES VACCINE

1. **Contents:** 1000 TCID 50 live attenuated measles virus (Schwarz) grown in chick embryo cells.
2. **Ideal age of initiating primary vaccination:** 9 months.
3. **Schedule of Primary vaccination :**
   Single dose if given beyond the age of 1 year. two doses if the first dose given before 9 months.
4. **Boosters:** Not recommended.
5. **When recommended:**
   Routine immunization.
   in epidemics & household contacts to be given between 6-9 months also.
6. **Dose:** 0.5 ml.
7. **Route of administration :** Subcutaneous.
8. **Site of administration:**
   Upper arm or anterolateral aspect of thigh.
9. **Preparation of site of administration:**
   Clean with antiseptic (spirit).
10. **Instructions to the mother after vaccination:**
    Mild fever & rash may appear after 5-7 days.
11. **Protection/efficacy:** Almost 95%
12. **Contra-indications :**
    1. Immunocompromised host.
    2. Severe (anaphylactic) egg allergy.
13. **Side effects:** fever and rash after 5-7 days.
14. **Complications :**
    Very rarely, subacute sclerosing panencephalitis.
15. **Storage at different levels and at doctor's clinic:**
    a) **When the vaccine is not is use:** 2°-8° C in the upper most compartment of refrigrator (together with diluent)
    b) **During immunization session.**
    On ice (within 1 hour of dissolving)
    c) **In case of electricity failure:** In an ice box.

MMR VACCINE

1. **Contents:** i) 1000 TCID - 50 live attenuated measles virus (Schwarz) grown on chick embryo cells)
   ii) 5000 TCID 50 live attenuated mumps (Urabe AM-9) cultured in embryonic hen egg.
   iii) 1000 TCID 50 live attenuated rubella (Wistar RA/3M) cultured on human diploid cells.
2. **Ideal age of initiating primary vaccination:** 15-18 months.
3. **Schedule of Primary vaccination :** Single dose.
4. **Boosters:** No recommended.
5. **When recommended:** Routine vaccination.
6. **Dose:** 0.5 ml.
7. **Route of administration :** Subcutaneous.
8. **Site of administration:** Upper arm or anterolateral aspect of thigh.
9. **Preparation of site of administration:** Clean with antiseptic (spirit).
10. **Instructions to the mother after vaccination:** Mild fever & rash may appear after 5-7 days.
11. **Protection/efficacy:** Almost 90-95%
12. **Contra-indications :** Immunocompromised host.
    - Severe egg allergy
    - Pregnancy.
13. **Side effects:**
    (i) Mild fever and rash may appear after 5-7 days.
    (ii) Rarely parotid swelling may appear after 10 days.
    (iii) Rarely arthralgia & mild lymphadenitis after 7-10 days.
14. **Complications :** As with measles.
15. **Storage at different levels and at doctor's clinic:**
    a) **When the vaccine is not is use :** 2-8 C in upper compartment of fridge (together with diluent)
    b) **During immunization session.** On ice (use within one hour of dissolving)
    c) **In case of electricity failure:** In ice box.

MEASLES / MMR VACCINE 6

Dr. Daya Sharma (DS) & Dr. Subhash Arya (SA)

Q.1. Measles vaccine is recommended to be given at the age of 9 months. Good number of children get measles before the age of 9 months. Why can't it be given at earlier age say at 5 to 6 months ?

DS : The measles vaccine can't be given at 5 to 6 months because of the poor serocoversion response at this age (upto 50-60%) as compared to 90% when given at 9 months or later. The passively acquired maternal antibodies against measles persist in infants upto 7-8 months of age which interfere with the successful take of the vaccine at earlier ages.

SA : A Child of 6 to 9 months of age should also be given measles vaccine. (i) during an epidemic (ii) during the measles season (usually January to May) or (iii) on exposure to a case of Measles (within 72 hours) These infants would however require a booster (Measles or MMR) between 15 to 18 months of age.

Q.2. It is feared that if a measles dose is given at an early age (< 7 months) and the child fails to seroconvert. then it may induce an immunological tolerance which would not allow seroconversion with subsequent dose of measles. Is it true ?

No, recent studies have clearly shown that the fear of immunological tolerance is unfounded.

Certain earlier studies had shown that those infants who had received measles vaccine at an early age ((i.e. in the presence of maternal antibodies) had an altered immunological response with subsequent dose of vaccine, resulting in low levels of antibody response. This led to a suspicion that early immunisation may lead to immunological tolerance. However more recent clinical studies (based on outbreak investigation) have clearly shown that revaccination of children, who had received vaccine earlier than 9-12 months, had produced adequate clinical protection even if they did not have adequate antibody response. Thus it seems that immunological tolerance in more a serological phenomenon rather than a clinically important phenomenon.

Q.3. If the measles vaccine is given at the right time (9 months) is there any need for repeating another dose ?

There is no need for repeating another dose of measles vaccine if the first dose is given at or after 9 months. The immunity persists for 15 years as has been shown by many prospective studies.

A booster of measles is not usually required after a primary dose of measles vaccine given at or after 9 months. However 10-15% of such children fail to seroconvert and may benefit from a second dose. If available MMR may be given at 15-18 months of age. Besides ensuring seroconversion against measles in those who failed to seroconvert with the first dose, it will also protect against Mumps and Rubella. See also Q. 13.

Q.4. Is there any need for repeating another dose of measles vaccine if it is given below the age of 9 months (if administered at 6 months of age)? if yes, then at what age repeat dose should be given. What is the ideal interval between two doses of measles vaccine?

DS : If the first dose is given at earlier than 9 months, then there is a need to revaccinate these children later at the age of 15-18 months (either Measles vaccine or as MMR).

SA : There is no ideal interval, as we are not boosting the vaccination but seroconverting those who failed to do so earlier. The second dose is given only after 15 months of age to ensure that all children do seroconvert.

Q.5. Now-a-days the recommendation is to give measles vaccine between 9-15 months of age. If a child does not get it within the specified time, can he get it later? Is there any upper age limit for giving measles vaccine ?

Yes, child can get measles vaccine later. There is no upper age limit for measles vaccination.

Q.6. UIP/EPI do not recommend MMR vaccine while this vaccine is being used widely in several developed countries of the world. What is the reason ?

The MMR vaccine is widely used in developed countries because the vaccine effectively reduces or eliminates congenital rubella syndrome as also mumps. Moreover the combination does not alter the immunogenecity of measles or other constitutents. UIP/EPI has not recommended MMR so far probably probably because of the economic and logistic constraints.

The Immunisation Advisory Committee of the Indian Academy of Pediatrics has recently recommended inclusion of MMR in the National immunization Programme.

Q.7. If economy is not the constraint, can measles vaccine be replaced by MMR to be given at the age of 9 months? Will second dose of MMR be required in such a situation?

MMR vaccine should only be given after the age of 1 year preferably at 15 months or later. Its effectiveness before 12 months is suspect. Also unlike measles, there is no compulsion to give mumps and rubella vaccine before that age, as these disease by and large do not occur in infancy unlike measles.

Q.8. Many pediatricians give a dose of measles at the age of 6-9 months, followed by a dose of MMR at the age of 15-18 months. What is your opinion regarding such a practice ?

DS : The measles vaccine should not be given routinely before 9 months of age because of poor seroconversion and thereby leave the child vulnerable for long period of 6 months or more at a time when the risk of measles is greatest.

SA : There is really not harm in giving measles vaccine at 6-9 months followed by MMR at 15 months.

First dose may be given before 9 months of age, only if a 2nd dose can be ensured after 15 months of age. This may be an acceptable procedure in an office practice, but this procedure may not be desirable at community level where large number of children may fail to return for the second dose.

Q.9. Why vaccine against measles is given at 15 months in USA but at 9 months of age in our country ? Are our children any different from those of USA ?

The age of vaccination is determined by two factors viz. decline in maternal antibody titres and the age of natural infection in developed countries (like USA the maternal antibodies decline by 9-12 months of age and most cases of measles occur after 5 years of age, so that a wide "window" is available for vaccination and hence the age of 15-18 months was selected as at that age more than 95% children got seroconverted.

On the other hand, maternal antibodies in children in developing countries like India, decline facter (by 6-8 months of age) and the measles infection also tend to occur very early. In fact about 25% cases of measles in our country occur less than 1 year of age and hence there is a need to protect children earlier tan 1 years. Studies has shown that one dose of measles vaccine at

9 months of age in developing countries also produce 85-90% seroconversion, and hence this age was choosen for immunising children in the UIP.

Q.10. What will happen if we give only one dose of measles vaccine at 6 months of age as we know that some cases of measles can occur even between 6-9 month of age ?

You are quite right that some cases (about 10% of all) can occur between 6-9 months of age but if we give presently available measles vaccine at 6 months, then only about 50% children would seroconverts. Other 50 would thus remain susceptible.

Q.11. What can be done to protect children below 9 months of age, in a routine manner ?

Actually in highly endemic countries like India, it may be desirable to follow two dose (first at 6 months and second at 15-18 month of age) schedule to ensure protection to maximum number of children. The immunization Advisory Committee of IAP has also recommended this schedule but the Govt. of India is reluctent to introduce it in the National health programme probably because of resource constraint and because of logistic difficulties.

Q.12. Can measles occur even after measles immunization ?

SA: Yes, Measles can occasionally occur even after measles vaccination.

DS: The reasons for suffering from measles after vaccination may be:

i) Immunisation at a very early age i.e. at 6 months or earlier.
ii) Use of expired or impotent vaccine.
iii) Not maintaining the proper cold chain and precautions
iv) True vaccine failures of around 10-15%

v) Simultaneous administration of immunoglobulins.
vi) Administration in immunosuppressed or congenitally immunodeficient individuals.

5-15% children fail to seroconvert after measles vaccine even when it is given at 9 months of age. A much larger number (upto 35%) may fail to react if the vaccine is given at 6 months of age. Children who fail to seroconvert would remain susceptible and may develop measles if exposed.

Apart from seroconversion, which have been studied under ideal situations, many workers in India have found a much lower clinical efficacy (47 to 69%) of single dose of measles vaccine at 9 months of age, in actual field situations. This may be due to por storage etc. of the vaccine. So in clinical practice it may not be very unusual to see child having measles after a dose of measles vaccine.

It should be remembered, however, that one dose of properly stored measles vaccine given after 15 months of age provides protection in more than 95% of cases. Compelling epidemiological factors (like frequent occurrence of severe measles in infancy) in our country has forced us to use this vaccine at 9 months, which is really not the absolute ideal age as far as the vaccine efficacy goes.

Q.13. In 1989, the committee on Infection Disease of American Academy of Pediatrics (AAP) and the Immunisation Practices advisory Committee (ACIP) in USA has recommended 2nd dose of Measles/MMR at school entry (4-6 yrs). What is the relevance of this recommendation to our country ?

In USA the age incidence of measls has shifted from 5-9 years in prevaccination era to 10-19 years at present time. This has happened after a very high rate of coverage for many years with one dose of measles vaccine. (Given as MMR at 15 months of age), introduced in USA in 1962. This late occurence of disease suggested waning of immunity in some cases and hence these bodies have recommended a booster at school entry.

In our country we are still struggling to achieve universal infants immunisation and to control the high incidence of early measles (in first years of age) which is often fatal. For the next few years our sole emphasis has to be on immunizing all children with one dose of measles so that the incidence of this dangerous disease can be largely controlled.

Hence these recommendation have no relevance in our country in the forseable future.

Q.14. Can adults be given measles vaccine, if they were not vaccinated in their childhood ?

Yes, if they have not already suffered from measles.

Although theoretically there is no objection in giving measles vaccine to an unvaccinated adult, however in practice it would be rarely required. Majority of individuals in our country, suffer from measles by 5 years of age and hence it would be difficult to find a suceptible individual after that age.

Q.15. A child has already suffered from doubtful measles. Should this child be given measles vaccine ?

Yes. There is no adverse reaction expected in such a case following vaccination.

Q.16. Is it advisable to give measles vaccination to a child who has suffered from measles in the past ?

DS : No, it is not indicated.

SA : Even the best of the clinicians have erred in diagnosing measles at times. In absence of a proof of seroconversion, I would recommend the vaccine strongly. Measles disease at any age is best avoided.

Q.17. Some parents believe that measles is inevitable and children should not be protected against this infection. What are your comments on this ?

They should be made to understand the morbidity & mortality caused by measles and its effective prevention by a timely administration of measles vaccine, which is highly effective and safe.

Example of small pox, which was also once considered inevitable, may be cited to convince the parents.

Q.18. What should be done to contacts of measles ? Recently measles vaccine is being recommended for prevention of measles in household contacts. What are your views on this? Will you prefer this over gammaglobulins?

Measles vaccine is recommended for prevention of measles in susceptible household contacts, only if it can be given within 72 hours of exposure. After that time only gammaglobulins are effective.

Q.19. If we decided to give immunoglobulin, which one should we prefer, measles specific gammaglobulin or nonspecific gammaglobulin? Kindly specify the dose also.

Measles specific immunoglobulin is definitely preferred over non specific immunoglobulin. However specific measles gammaglobulin is not presently available in our country.

The dose of usually available 16.5% (non-specific) gammaglobulins is 0.06ml/kg given intramuscularly.

This must be given within 6 days of exposure to be really effective.

Q.20. A 3 months old infant is in contact with his elder sibling who is suffering from measles. Does this child need prevention ?

No, Infants upto 5-6 months of age have adequate levels of maternally derived measles antibodies which protect them against the disease and hence such infants do not need any immunoglobulins or vaccine for protection.

Q.21. Can we give measles vaccine and immunoglobulin concurrently to prevent measles in a household contact ?

No, they can not be given together, as immunoglobulin would interfere with measles uptake.

Q.22. If immunoglobulin was preferred for the prevention of measles, how soon should the measles vaccine be given to this child ?

Measles vaccine should be given at least 6 weeks and preferably after 12 weeks of the administration of immunoglobulins.

Q.23. There has been a fear that if immunoglobulins are given (for prevention of measles) during prodrome of measles, it can precipitate encephalitis. Is it true ?

No, it does not precipitate encephalitis.

Q.24. Is the incidence of SSPE higher among vaccinated children compared to naturally infected children ?

No, on the contrary the incidence of SSPE is quite low in vaccinated children as compared to naturally infected children. It is 0.1/100,00 vaccinees as against 0.5 - 2/100,000 infected persons.

The use of measles vaccine has dramatically decreased the incidence of SSPE in USA. Further epidemiological data has not suggested any casual relationship between measles vaccine and SSPE.

Q.25. What will happen if measles vaccine is given in the prodrome of measles ?

The Measles vaccine is neither effective nor harmful if given in the prodrome of measles.

Q.26. Can measles vaccine prevent chicken pox ?

No, it does not prevent chicken pox.

Q.27. How soon can the measles vaccine be given after an attack of chicken pox ?

It can be given 3-6 weeks after an attack of chicken pox.

Q.28. Are any special precautions necessary while diluting a measles vaccine ?

Yes, the following precautions should be taken while diluting the measles vaccine :

i) The diluent also must have been kept at 2-8° C (with vaccine).
ii) It should not be done under direct sunlight.
iii) Care should be taken to avoid spilling (in case of ampoules).
iv) It should not be shaken vigorously after dilution.

Q.29. What is the diluent of measles vaccine? Can we dissolve it in distilled water ?

DS : Yes, it can be dissolved in sterile distilled water.
SA : The diluent used is buffered distiled water.

Q.30. Manufacturer (SII) provides instructions with the diluent, indicating that it should not be frozen. What is the reason ?

DS : The diluent should not be frozen because it has to be used in liquid form. To bring it into the liquid state, it will have to be warmed up or kept at room temperature for a long time and this interferes with the potency of the vaccine.

SA : Freezing may also destroy the buffer in the diluent.

Manufacturers inform that the ampoule should not be frozen as it may develop cracks.

Q.31. In which shelf of refrigerator, measles vaccine should be stored ?

It should be stored in the uppermost shelf of the refrigerator or in the chiller tray together with BCG ampoules.

Q.32. For how long can the diluted vaccine be kept and at what temperature ?

The diluted vaccine should be kept at +2° to + 8°C for 3-4 hrs only; though the present heat stable vaccine after reconstitution retain potency for upto 24 hours at 4° to 8°C.

Q.33. It is mentioned in the instructions that vaccine should not be shaken vigorously after dilution, what is the harm ?

Vigorous shaking should be avoided as it may lead to frothing and scum formation which will interfere with the accurate measurement of the dose.

Q.34. Can measles vaccine be given to children with known egg allergy ?

DS : No, it is contraindicated in cases of known egg allergy.

SA : If there is an history of anaphylactic reaction to egg (urticaria with hypotension or difficult in breathing or hoarseness) then it should not be given without prior skin testing. Scratch testing should be done, with 1:10 dilution followed by intradermal test 1:100 dilution of the measles vaccine. However, milder forms of egg allergy is not a contraindication for measles vaccination.

Q.35. Is it really necessary to introduce egg before giving measles vaccine ?

No

Although it is true that children allergic to eggs may have adverse reactions to measles vaccine as it is grown on chick embryo fibroblasts, yet introduction of eggs (prior to vaccinations) is not necessary. This is because reactions to measles vaccine are seen only in those individuals who have Type I allergic (anaphylactic) reactions to eggs which is extremely rare (less than 1 per 100,000 population).

Q.36. You have said that measles vaccine should not be given to children who are allergic to egg. Many of our families are strictly vegetarian. Can I give measles vaccine to the children of such families also without being able to initiate egg feeds in them? Can I do a sensitivity test?

Yes, it can be given and there is not need to do sensitivity test in such children, as explained above.

Presently available SII measles vaccine is grown on Human Diploid cells and hence causes no allergic reactions.

Q.37. It is said two live virus vaccines should not be given concurrently. Can measles vaccine be given with polio vaccine ?

Yes, measles vaccine can be given with polio vaccine. (See also Chapter 1 on General consideration)

Q.38. Can BCG and measles vaccine be given concurrently ?

Simultaneous administration of BCG and measles vaccine should preferably be avoided as measles vaccine depresses the cell mediated immune response which may interfere with the successful uptake of BCG.

There is no authentic study which has substantiated decreased uptake of BCG or shown any harmful effect of such a practice.

Q.39. A 9 months old child is receiving post-exposure rabies prophylaxis. Can this child be given measles vaccine ?

Yes, this child be given measles vaccine.

Q.40. Can measles vaccine be given to children on long term steroids or on chemotherapy (compromised hosts) ?

DS : No, measles vaccine should not be given to a child on long term steroids or chemotherapy. It should only be given after a minimum period of 3 months and 6 months of discontinution of steroids or chemotherapy respectively.

SA : Short term (<2 weeks) or alternate day steroids are not a contraindication to measles vaccine.

Q.41. What are the absolute contraindications of measles vaccine ?

The absolute contraindication are :

i) Leukemia, Hodgkin's disease or other malignant conditions.
ii) Congenital immunodeficiency states.
iii) Acute illnesses or active tuberculosis.
iv) Anaphylactic sensitivity to hen's egg or neomycin.
v) Pregnant women.

On theoritical grounds measles vaccine should not be administered to pregnant women. However measles vaccine virus has not been shown to cross the placenta and infect the foetus.

Q.42. What site should be selected for measles vaccine administration and how to prepare the site for injection?

it is given at anterolateral aspect of thigh or at upper shoulder by subcutaneous route. The site should be cleaned with spirit or alcohol but is allowed to dry before vaccination.

Q.43. Should vigorous rubbing be done at the site of injection after measles vaccination ?

No.

Q.44. Should hot fomentation be done at the site of injection ?

No, there is no need.

Q.45. Accidentally I have injected measles vaccine through intramuscular route instead of subcutaneous route. Will the side effects be more ?

No, it can be given safely by I.M. route also.

Q.46. Can antiseptics like spirit be used for cleaning the site of injection? Would it have harmful effects on the potency of vaccine as the measles vaccine is a live virus vaccine ?

Yes, spirit can be used, However, it must be allowed to dry completely before vaccination otherwise measles vaccine is likely to be inactivated.

Q.47. Can measles vaccine be given to a child who has received blood transfusion a week back?

Ideally measles vaccine should not be given for upto 6 weeks following a blood transfusion.

Q.48. Can measles vaccine be given to a child with active tuberculosis ?

No, it should not be given to a child with active tuberculosis as it may further flare up the disease.

Q.49. Can measles vaccine be given to a child who is case of pulmonary tuberculosis and has received antituberculous treatment for 3 months ?

Yes, it can now be safely given.

Q.50. In a country like ours where tuberculosis is an endemic disease, is it necessary to do a Mantoux test before giving measles vaccine ?

No it is not necessary to do Mantoux prior to measles vaccine as measles vaccine has not been shown to exacerebate tuberculosis.

Q.51. After measles vaccination some children develop measles like rash after 7-10 days of inoculation. Does this indicate good immunity?

No, there is no such corelation.

Development of measles like rash after vaccine is seen as a side effect in only 7 out of 1000 vaccinated children. It has no correlation with immunity.

Q.52. What are the clinical manifestation of measles in an immunised child ?

Measles in these cases usually occurs in a modified (attenuated) form with somewhat longer incubation period and milder clinical symptoms of fever, rash, corryza etc. On the other hand earlier atypical measles occured among those children who had previously been vaccinated with killed measles vaccine in USA. This was a sort of hypersensitive reaction with high fever, atypical rash (starting from hand & feet and spreding centrally), pleural effusion etc. This is not seen in India as killed vaccine has never been used here.

Q.53. A child has developed parotid swelling after 10 days of inoculation of MMR. Could it be due to the vaccine ?

It is most likely a side-effect of mumps vaccination. The parotitis following mumps vaccine occurring between 7 to 14 days, is a known complication of mumps vaccine.

Q.54. Can MMR vaccine be given to children who already have had mumps in the past ?

DS : Yes, it can be given.

SA : Parotitis itself can have different etiologies besides being confused with lymphadenitis. Thus MMR should be given even if the child gives a history of parotid swellings. MMR will also provide protection against measles and rubella and would not harm even if the child actually had had mumps in the past.

Q.55. What should be done to the contacts of mumps ? Can MMR vaccine or immunoglobulin help in this situation ?

The vaccine may help, if given within a day of contact with mumps patients. There is no harm even if it is given in prodromal period but it is unlikely to be effective. The role of immunoglobulin is yet to be proven convincingly.

Q.56. "MMR should only be given to female children" What is your opinion on this statement ?

Rubella vaccine alone may be required only in female children but MMR vaccine should be given to both male and female children as mumps is an important disease in both the sexes.

Q.57. Rubella vaccine is given at the age of 1-2 years in USA and at adolescence in UK. In your opinion which is the right practice ?

MMR should be given at 1-2 yrs of age to decrease the incidence of congenital rubella effectively and not at adolescent age as in UK; as theat would not prevent the transmission cycle completely.

Rubella, usually a very mild disease, causes congenital anomalies in the fetus when it occurs in pregnant females. So really speaking, the only time rubella needs to be prevented in at child bearing age. In United Kingdom the policy of immunising (seronegative) adolescent females is followed only for this reason, so that the vaccine is not unnecessarily wasted.

However, seroconversion after a singly dose of Rubella vaccine (either alone or as MMR) at 15-18 months of age probably provides life long immunity to all children. It also helps to provide herd immunity and thus to prevent transmission of rubella in the community. Further it is far easier to vaccinate children at 15-18 months of age rather than adolescent girls. Hence USA follows the policy of giving MMR at 15-18 months of age. However recent data from USA suggests that this policy has failed to decrease the incidence of congenital rubella syndrome and hence they have started vaccination of susceptible adole scents also.

This controversy is irelevant at present, as the incidence of congenital rubella syndrome in our country is extremely low and more than 90% of child bearing age group women have protective antibodies against Rubella.

Q.58. As rubella vaccine is not available in isolated form; can adolescent girls be given MMR vaccine for protection against rubella, who have not received the same in their childhood?

Yes, no harm will be done if they receive measles and mumps vaccine also together with rubella.

Q.59. Can MMR (for rubella) be given to married women? What should be the minimum interval between receiving rubella vaccine (or MMR in our country) and time of conceiving ?

Yes, rubella vaccine or MMR can be given to (seronegative) married women who are not pregnant, but they should be told to avoid pregnancy during next 3-4 months.

Traditionally fears have been expressed of possible teratogenic effects of rubella vaccine in pregnancy. However since the introduction of vaccine 20 years back, more than 200 pregnant women in USA have accidently received rubella vaccine and on follow up none of the offsprings developed teratogenicity. However pregnancy remains a contraindication to rubella vaccine but accidental rubella vaccination in unsuspected pregnancy is not an indication for termination of pregnancy. Routine pregnancy testing is not to be ordered, if the history of pregnancy is denied by the woman.

Q.60. Recently a strain of rubella virus has been used as nasal spray vaccine. How effective is this and is this curently available ?

The strain RA-27 can be given by nasal spray and it is more than 95% effective in providing immunity against rubella. It is not yet available in India.

This mode of vaccination is not yet recommended for routine use.

Q.61. It is said that two live virus vaccines can not be given simultaneously but in MMR there are three live virus vaccines being given concurrently. Do they not interfere in development of immunity of each other ?

DS : No, they do not interefere with the development of immunity of each other. The seroconversion rates for all the three components exceeds more than 90%.

SA : MMR can be given with other live virus vaccine (OPV) also.

Different live virus vaccine do not interfere with development of immunity against each other as long as they are given on the same day. If by any chance they can not be given on the same day then an interval of at least 4 weeks should be kept to evoke desirable immune response.

Q.62. What are the contraindications of MMR vaccine?

Same as any other live virus vaccine (as measles) ref: Q.41, of this chapter.

Q.63. Rubella is a live virus vaccine and when given to a host is liable to be activated and become communicable to the close contact of vaccinee. Does it mean that we avoid giving MMR (rubella) to a child whose mother or women contacts are known to be pregnant ?

No, vaccinated children do not transmit the infection to their close contacts.

Some vaccinees may shed small amount of virus from pharynx, 7 to 28 days after vaccination, but vaccine virus is not transmissable to susceptible contacts. In any case fears of teratogancity of rubella vaccine virus have been allayed (supra)

Q.64. What are the complications of measles and MMR vaccines?

Side effects are few and mild in the form of fever and rash which appear at about 8th day of vaccination. Cough, coryza and pharyngits may also occur. Febrile convulsions may rarely accompany the fever. Severe reations are uncommon. (Table 1)

Table 1
Reactions to measles vaccine.

Major Reactions	*Rates/100,000*
Encephalitis/Encephalopathy	*0.1*
SSPE	*0.05 - 0.1*
Convulsions	*0.02 - 1.9*
Death	*0.02 to 0.3*
Minor Reactions	*Rates/100*
Fever	*8.3*
Diarrhea	*3.0*
Catarrh	*0.95*
Rash	*0.7*

NB. Rubella vaccine in MMR may cause arthralgia while mumps component may lead to parotitis.

Q.65. Which other vaccines can be administered with measles/MMR vaccine and which vaccines should not be administered concurrently?

DPT and OPV can be given with Measles or MMR vaccine.

Also Hepatitis B and typhoid can be given with measles vaccine if indicated. There is no contraindication for any of the currently available vaccine to be given together with measles vaccine. (except BCG which is preferably avoided).

Q.66. Are facilities of rubella antibody estimation available in Delhi & other parts of our country?

Yes, they are available in India at many centres. In Delhi they are available at NICD, AIIMS and MAMC

Q.67. Kindly comment on aerosolized measles vaccine?

Recently many studies have indicated the effectiveness of aerosolized vaccine in infants as young as 4-6 months old. The strain used is Edmonston-Zagreb human diploid cells strain. The vaccine is effective in young infants as respiratory epithelium has only secretory IgA and no IgG, which intereferes with the final immunity achieved. But the equipment and procedure is combersome for field conditions and as such it is not recommended at present.

Same strain has now been used as sub cutanous injection with encouraging results.

Q.68. Is'nt there some way by which we can even actively immunize young infants against measles ?

Recent development of Edmonston Zagreb strain of measles vaccine holds some hope of protecting even young infants (less than 6 months of age) with measles vaccine. Studies utilising high potency EZ strain have shown that it is effective in producting seroconversion even in young infants. WHO has also recently (1990) recommended the use of this vaccine in developing countries at 4-6 months of age. Presently SII is supplying a vaccine which contains 5000 IU of EZ strain of measles virus grown on Human diploid cells. This can be given to infants between 6-9 months of age but is not sufficiently potent for infants less than 6 months of age when one requires 10 to 25,000 IU of EZ strain.

Bibliography

1. Aggarwal SK : Study of passive measles immunity in the first year of life and seroconversion responses following vaccinations at 6-12 months of age. Thesis submitted for the degree of Medicine (Pediatrics) at Univ. of Delhi, 1988.
2. Andre FE. Thermodegradation of lyophilized measles vaccine. Review of Infect. Dis. Vol. 5, 1984.
3. British Research Committee: Third report on Vaccination against measles, clinical trial of live measles vaccine given alone and live vaccine preceeded by killed vaccine. Practitioner, 1971, 206: 458-466.

4. Campbell AG: Immunization for the immunosuppressed child. Arch of Dis. in child. 1988, 63: 113-114.
5. Centers for Disease Control : Measles prevention : Recommendation of the Immunization Practices Advisory Committee (ACIP). MMWR 1989, 38:S-9.
6. Centre for diseases control, Recommendations of the Immunization Protection Advisory Committee: Measles prevention, MMWR, 31:217-231.
7. Cherian S; Measles, In: Immunization Practices in children: Indian Academy of Pediatrics (Delhi), 1988, Editors, A Datta, S. K. Mittal and V. Agarwal pp 43-57.
8. Collaborative Study by the Ministry of Health Kenya and the World Health Organization: Measles immunity in the first year of life and the optimum age of vaccination in Kenyan children. Bull WHO 1982, 57:89.
9. Davis RM, Whitman ED, Orenstein WA, et al: A persistent outbreak of measles despite apprepriate control measures. Am J Epidemio 1987, 126: 438.
10. DGHS Measles Immunization Project, New Delhi, Nirman Bhawan, 1981.
11. Expanded Progamme on Immunization, Global Advisory Group. Weekly Epidemiol Rep. 1990, 65 : 5.
12. Ghosh S. Dhatt PS: Complications of measles, Ind. J Ch. Health, 1961, 10: 111-119.
13. Halsey NA, Boulos R, Mode F, Andre J, Bowan L, Yaegar RG, Toureau S, Rohde J, Boulos C, : Response to measles vaccine in Haitian infants 6-12 months old. Influence of maternal antibodies, malnutriation and concomittant illness. N.Engl. J. Med. 1985, 313: 544-549.
14. Job JS, John TJ, Joseph A: Antibody responses to measles immunization in India, Bull WHO, 1984, 62 : 737-741.
15. John TJ et al: Epidemiology and prevention of measles in rural South India, Ind J of Med Res. 1980, 72: 153-158.
16. Krugman S: Further attenuated measles vaccine: Characteristics and use. Rev of Inf. Dis, 1983, 5: 477-481.
17. Krugman S: Present status of measles and Rubella Immunization in the United States, A Medical Prog. Report, J.Ped. 1971, 78 : 1-14.

18. Krugman S: Present Status of measles and rubella immunization in the United States. A medical progress report. J Pediatr 1977, 90:1.
19. Krugman S, Giles JP, Friedma H, Stones SL Studies on immunity to measles. J Pediatr 1965, 66: 471.
20. Lerman SL, Bellinger M, brunkem JM: Clinical and serologic evaluation of measles, mumps and rubella (HPV-77:DE5 and RA 27/3) Virus vaccines, singly and in combination. Pediatrics 1981, 68:18.
21. Linnemann CC Jr, Dine MS, Rosella GA, et al: Measles immunity after revaccination: Results in children vaccined before 10 months of age. Pediatrics 1982, 69:332.
22. Loenning WKK, Coovadia HN: Age specific occurence rate of measles in Urban, peri-urban and rural environment, implications for time of vaccination, Lancet, 1983, 2, 324-326.
23. Manmohan et al : Optium age of measles immunization, Ind Ped. 1981, 18 : 631-635.
24. Markewitz LE, Sepulvedax J, Diaz-Ortega JL, et al: Immunization of six month old infant with different doses of Edmonston-Zagreb and Schwarz mealses vaccines. N Engl J Med 1990, 322:580.
25. Mehta M et al : Sero epidemiology of measles in Bombay. India J of Med Res 1972, 60:661.
26. Modlin JF, Jabbour JT, Titte JJ, et al: Epidemiologic studies of measles, measles vaccine, and subacute sclerosing panencephalitis. Pediatrics 1977, 59 : 505.
27. Pelota H, Heinonen O: Frequency of true adverse reactions: Measles-mumps-rebella vaccine. Lancet 1986, 1:939.
28. Saha SM et al : Seroconversion in different age groups after measles vaccination. Ind J Ped, 1985, 52 : 303-305.
29. Shasby DM, Shope TC, Dewns H, et al: Epidemic measles in a highly vaccinated population, N Engl J Med 1977, 296:585.
30. Sinha WP: Measles in children under 6 month of age: An epideminological study, J. Trop Ped., 1981, 27: 120-122.
31. Stetler HC, Orenstein WA, Bernier RH, et al: Impact of revaccination on children who initially received measles vaccine before 10 months of age. Pediatrics 1986, 77:47.
32. Sundervali MC et al : Post measles complications in infants and children. Ind Ped., 1979, 16, 437-439.

33. Tidjani O, Grunitsky B, Buerin N, et al: Serological effects of Edmonston-Zagerb, Schwarz and AIL-C measles vaccine strains given at ages 4-5 or 8-10 months. Lancet 1989, 2:1357.
34. Universal immunization programme: Manage cold chain system. A Manual: Ministry of Health & FW, Govt of India, New Delhi, 1987.
35. Whittle HC, Rowland NGM, Mann GF, Lamb WH & Lewis RA: Immunization of 4-6 months old Gambian infants with Edmonston-Zagreb measles vaccine. Lancet, 1984, 2: 834-837.
36. Whittle HC, Mann G, Eccles M, et al: Effects of dose and strain of vaccine on success of measles vaccination of infants aged 4-5 months. Lancet 1988, 1:963.
37. WHO Techn. Report Series: Measles vaccination, No. 693, 1983.
38. Vaccines used in EPI:Indications & Contraindication. Chronicle 1984,38:95-98, Abstracted form Bulletin WHO,1984,62:357-366.
39. Yeager AS, Davis JH et al: Measles immunization-successes and failures. J.A.M.A., 1977, 237-347.

TYPHOID VACCINE

1. **Contents:*** Contains *Salmonella typhi* 1000 million heat killed phenolized or acetone killed (AKD) bacteria per ml.
2. **Ideal age of initiating primary vaccination:** 2 years
3. **Schedule of Primary vaccination.** Two doses 4 weeks apart.
4. **Boosters:** Every 3 years.
5. **When recommended:** Routine immunization.
6. **Dose:** 0.25ml in <10 years.
0.5 ml in >10 years.
7. **Route of administration :** Subcutaneous.
8. **Site of administration:** Anterolateral aspect of thigh.
9. **Preparation of site of administration:** Clean with antiseptic (spirit).
10. **Instructions to the mother after vaccination:** To give antipyretic (paracetamol) in case of fever.
11. **Protection/efficacy:** 51-73% with phenolized vaccine, 70-94% with AKD
12. **Contra-indications :** None.
13. **Side effects:** Fever, local pain, malaise, headache, chills.
14. **Complications :** None.
15. **Storage at different levels and at doctor's clinic:**
    a) **When the vaccine is not is use :** In lowermost compartment of fridge (DO NOT FREEZE)
    b) **During immunization session.** Can be kept at room temperature.
    c) **In case of electricity failure:** Keep at cool & dark place.

* Combined Typhoid and Paratyphoid (TAB) is now not available.

TYPHOID VACCINE 7

Dr. Vijay Aggarwal (VA) & Dr. Raju Shah (RS)

Q.1. All gram negative bacteria vaccine make poor vaccines. How far is this statement correct ?

RS: Yes, all Gram negative bacterial vaccine are rather poor vaccines.

VA: In fact all bacteria (because of multiple antigenic determinants) make poor vaccines and not Gram negative bacteria in particular. This can also be inferred from the fact that life-long immunity following bacterial infections is rare. There are as many vaccines (if not more) against Gram negative organisms as against Gram positive ones.

Vaccines against Menigococci (Gr. A & C) and H. Influenzae b. are also vaccines against Gram negative organisms, but are fairly effective if given after the age of 2 years.

Q.2. What is the efficacy of presently available typhoid vaccines ? Are any of these vaccines effective enough to be given routinely ?

Presently, Typhoid (monovalent) and TA (Typhoid & paratyphoid A) vaccines are available in our country. They are available as heat killed phenolised vaccines or acetone killed and dried vaccines (AKD). Efficacy of these vaccines to protect against *Salmonella typhi* in various studies has ranged from 51% to 73% in case of phenolised and 70 to 94% in case of AKD vaccines.

In relation to efficacy of typhoid vaccines it should be remembered that protection achieved is partial as it can be overcome by larger inoculum of the infecting dose.

Average efficacy of phenol killed vaccine is about 50% while that of AKD vaccine is about 75%. However the efficacy of later vaccine in young children has never been shown. In USA AKD vaccine has been used only for Military personnel till now and not for children.

Q.3. Previously TAB vaccine used to be available. Now only monovalent typhoid vaccine is available. Are the side effects of monovalent vaccine lesser ?

Monovalent typhoid vaccine should be preferred because :

a) Not much is known about the efficacy of paratyphoid A component of TA or TAB vaccine.

b) Paratyphoid B is epidemiologically not important in our county.

c) Side effects of monovalent vaccine are less.

Q.4. The recent recommendation is to give typhoid vaccine above the age of 5 years. Has the incidence of typhoid fever dropped sufficiently enough in children less than 5 years to justify its use beyond this age only ? Or is it that the vaccine is not effective before the age of 5 years ?

There is enough evidence from the review of the recent epidemiological data that 20% cases of typhoid occur below the age of 5 years in our country. In a recent National Workshop, the Indian Academy of Pediatrics (IAP) recommended that the the age of starting typhoid vaccination should be 2 years, although the vaccine is probably effective even at 6 months of age.

Immunization of children less than 6 years should be done only with Phenol killed vaccine as AKD vaccine is not effective.

Q.5. What is the schedule of typhoid vaccine. The manufacturers recommend two doses at an interval of 15 days. Do you agree with this ?

Schedule of typhoid vaccine as suggested by IAP is to start vaccination at 2 years and give 0.25 ml of the vaccine subcutaneously at 4 weeks interval. Booster vaccinations are given every 3 yearly.

The recommendation of the manufacturer to give doses at 2 weeks interval is not basically wrong, as an interval of 2 to 4 weeks has been used in various studies. American Academy of Pediatrics recommends 3 wks interval.

Immunologically 4 weeks interval in superior. Lesser intervals should be used only in case of epidemics or family contacts.

Q.6. Does the dose of vaccine vary at different ages ?

The dose of the vaccine does vary according to the age. Children below 10 years are given 0.25ml (250 million bacilli) While those above 10 years are given 0.5 ml of the vaccine. (Recommendations AAP, 1989).

Q.7. How can the children be protected from typhoid fever in case of an epidemic ?

Protection from typhoid fever can be achieved by :–

i) Safe drinking water and hygienic food preparation.
ii) Adopting proper sanitation methods for excreta disposal.
iii) Education regarding hand washing and personal hygiene.
iv) Vaccination against typhoid: Initial 2 doses may be given at 2 to 3 wks interval rather than 4 wks interval.

Some authorities recommend 3 doses at 1 wk interval but the ultimate protection provided may be less than 2 doses at 3 wks interval.

Q.8. Now acetone killed vaccine is also available. What are the advantages of this vaccine over phenolized vaccine ?

Main advantage of AKD vaccine is the better efficacy of this type of vaccine as explained in Q.2. The duration of protection is longer than with phenolised vaccine and even one dose provides significant protection especially in endemic areas. Acetone killed vaccine retains some of the Vi antigen which may account for some of the differences.

Efficacy of AKD vaccine in young children has never been proven.

Q.9. Can typhoid vaccine be given through intradermal route ? Can AKD vaccine be also given intradermally ?

Phenolised typhoid vaccine can be given through intradermal route 0.1 ml. vaccine give intradermally provides as strong an antibody response as the larger dose given subcutaneously. Data on protective effect of this route, in field trials, is however lacking. Intradermal injection of AKD vaccine is associated with more side effects than phenolised vaccine and is not recommended by American Academy of Pediatrics.

Q.10. Despite the fact that the AKD vaccine is more effective than phenol killed vaccine, why is it that only the latter vaccine is available for routine use ? Is there any technical problem in manufacturing AKD vaccine ?

This matter should be taken up with the manufacturers because even in U.S.A., AKD vaccine is available only to military personnel and only the heat-phenol inactivated vaccine is available commercially.

Q.11. What prophylaxis should be given to household contacts of typhoid patient ?

Same as explained in Q.7. In addition, the index case should be followed up to to see that he is not becoming a chronic carrier.

Q.12. Two types of typhoid vaccines are available viz child and adult vaccine. What is the difference between the two ?

RS : The two vaccines differ from each other in the number of killed bacilli they contain per dose:

Child vaccine : *Salm Typhi 330* million, *paratyphi A* 160 million

Adult vaccine: *Salm typhi* 1000 million, *paratyphi A* 500 million.

VA: Child and adult vaccines are probably not available any more.

The doses mentioned in Q.6 pertain to the adult type of vaccine.

Q.13. Can typhoid vaccine be given to children less than two year old in epidemic situations ?

Yes, Phenolised vaccine can and should be given to children above 6 months of age in epidemic situations.

Q.14. How often should the booster doses be given?

Typhoid vaccine needs to be repeated every 3 years.

Q.15. What changes are reflected in Widal test after typhoid vaccine administration ? How do these changes differ from those affected by an attack of typhoid fever ?

Following an innoculation with typhoid vaccine the H agglutinis rise and may persist for year. While the O agglutinins are also formed but do not reach as high as H agglutinin titres and also do not persist for more than a few months. With infection also, both O and H titres rise. Rise of O titres is more pronounced but short lived.

In infection also the response of 'H" agglutinins is brisker and more marked compared to O agglutinins. Usually the rise in agglutinin titres (O & H) following natural infection are rather short lived probably because of antimicrobial therapy. In clinical practice it may be difficult to distinguish whether a rise in O & H titres are due to previous vaccine or due to natural infection. Clinical picture, intensity of rise in O and H titres and the history and time elapsed since vaccination, may help in distinguishing widal reaction of natural infection from that due to vaccine.

Q.16. Can widal test be used to know the efficacy of typhoid vaccine ?

Although widal test does show rise in titres as explained above, but efficacy & potency of typhoid vaccine can not be judged by this test because these antibodies (anti H & anti O) have poor correlation with efficacy & potency of typhoid vaccine.

Efficacy of Typhoid vaccine is better judged by Vi antibody levels.

Q.17. Should typhoid vaccine be given to children who have already suffered from typhoid fever ?

The development of immunity following natural infection is there but unfortunately it is not so in all the cases. Use of antibiotics may also inhibit the development of immune response. So, the children recovering from typhoid should be given a vaccine like any other child to prevent re-infection.

This can be given only after 2-3 months of recovery.

Q.18. Till what age should typhoid vaccine be given?

There is no upper age limit for typhoid vaccine.

Q.19. What are the side effects of typhoid vaccine ?

Side effects of typhoid vaccine include systemic (fever, malaise,headache) and local reactions (erythema, induration, pain). Side effects are least with intradermal vaccination with phenolised vaccine.

Q.20 What are the contraindications to typhoid vaccination ?

Acute febrile illness is the only contra-indication to the use of typhoid vaccine.

Q.21. Can typhoid and cholera vaccine be given simultaneously ?

Yes. But practically there is no need to combine typhoid with cholera vaccine.

Q.22. A live oral typhoid vaccine is being currently used in field trials. Kindly throw some light on this vaccine.

A live oral typhoid vaccine has been tried in large number of field trials in Chile, Egypt, Indonesia etc. For this vaccine Ty21a strain of *Salm typhi* has been used. This is a mutant strain which lacks the enzyme UDP-galactose-4-epimerase. This enzyme is responsible for incorporation of galactose into cell-wall polysaccharide, through a series of intermediary metabolic steps. While the galactose present in the intestine can be accumulated in the cell wall of the organism, but the same in the absence of this epimerase, cannot be converted into polysaccharide. Accumulation of intermediary products of galactose in the cells cause disruption of cell membrane and ultimately cell lysis. Continued faulty boisynthesis of cell wall polysaccharide provides immune effect while subsequent bacterial lysis accounts for low virulence of this strain.

At least I billion organisms of *Salm typhi Ty21a* are available in each capsule of this vaccine. The vaccine strain has been shown to be safe, protective and amenable to mass vacination when formulated in enteric coated capsules.

Oral typhoid vaccine prepared form Ty 21a strain, is now available in USA under the trade name of Vivotif Berna (Manufactureed in Switzerland). Dosage is I capsule to be swallowed 1 hour before meals with cold drinks on days 1, 3, 5 and 7. Capsule should not be chewed. It is as effective as injectiable vaccine with much less side effects. Side effects which may be noticed are nausea, vomiting and abdominal cramps. The need for booster for this vaccine has not yet been determined.

Q.23. Are there any disadvantages of oral typhoid vaccine ?

Yes, oral typhoid vaccine cannot be used in children less than 6 years of age, as it is available in capsule form. Also it should not be used with oral antibioties or sulfa drugs or when the patient has a febrile illness or a gastrointestinal illness. Oral typhoid vaccine, being a new research product, is still quite costly. Also multiple doses are required and the duration of protection offered is not yet certain.

Q.24. Is any other typhoid vaccine likely to be available in near future which maybe given to children also ?

Yes, another injectable typhoid vaccine which incorporates attenuated Vi antigen has recently become available. This vaccine is prepared by attenuating the virulent Vi antigen which is associated with cell wall polysaccharide of *Salm. typhi.* At least two vaccines utilizing Vi antigen have been sanctioned for trial. Preliminary trials have been carried out in Nepal, South Africa, Indonesia etc. and have shown promising results. Its efficacy is near 80%. This vaccine may soon be sanctioned for general use.

Q.25. Recently, the Govt. of India has discontinued the routine use of typhoid vaccine in the national immunization programme. What is the reason for the same ? What shall I tell my patient who demands typhoid vaccine for his child ?

The reasons forwarded by an expert committee which recommended discontinuance of typhoid vaccine in EPI programme were :

i) Information on the epidemiology of enteric fever in different parts of the country is inadequate and even the size of problems is not adequately known.
ii) In a limited study in the urban slums of Delhi, it was found that less than 1% of the children get this disease each year.
iii) The conventional type of vaccine used was affording a protection range of 51-73%. The protection provided was also not absolute.
iv) The use of vaccine is associated with local and constitutional side reactions and therefore there is general resistance on the part of children to accept it and as a result the performance in EPI has been consistently low.
v) Acetone killed vaccine trials may be conducted by ICMR in India and depending on the outcome, its use in public health practice could be reviewed.

If the parents demand conventional typhoid vaccine, you may still give it after explaining the limited efficacy & possible side effects of the vaccine. Govt. of India has also recommended the use of typhoid vaccine on demand.

Bibliography

1. Bart KJ et al Vaccine preventable disease in developing world, PCNA, 1990, 37:733-763.
2. Centres for Disease Control : Health Information for International Travel, 1989. HHS Publication No. (CDC) 89-8280, July, 1989.

3. Feigin RD. Infections due to *Salmonella*, In Nelson's Text Book of Pediatries XIII Edition, p. 600 W.B. Saunders Philadephia. U.S.A. 1987.
4. Germanier R. New Vaccines against typhoid fever. World Pediatrics and Child Care 1987:3:155-126.
5. Jool. Present status and prespectives of vaccination against typhoid fever. In: Proceedings of the International Conference on the application of vaccines against viral, Rickettssial and Bacterial diseases of men, 1970. Washington D.C. Pan American Organisation (Sci Publ. No. 226): 329-341.
6. Levine MM, Black RE, Feneccio C et al. Chilean Typhoid Commission. Interventions to control endemic typhoid fever: Field studies in Santiago Chile. In: Control and eradication of infectious diseases an international symposium. Pan American Health Organisation. Co. publication series No. 1 PAHO Washington DC 1985; 37-53.
7. Levine MM. New Vaccines against Typhoid fever. World Pediatrics and Child care 1987, 3: 115-126.
8. Levine MM, Ferraccio, C, Black RE et al: Progress in vaccines against typhoid fever. Rev Infect Dis II 1989, (Suppl 3): S552.
9. Morton S.W. Vaccine For Foreign traval PCNA 1990, 37:757-769.
10. Mullighan TO. Typhoid fever in young children. BMJ 1971; 41:665-7.
11. Patnaik KC, Kapoor PN. A note on the incidence of typhoid in Delhi, IJMR 1957, 55: 228-39.
12. Ryan CA, Hargrett-Bean NT, Blake PA: *Salmonella typhi* infections in the United States 1975-1984: Increasing role of foreign travel. Rev Infect Dis 1989, II:I.
13. Saili A. Typhoid in Immunisation Practices in children. Ed. A Datta,SK Mittal and V Agarwal. Ind. Acd pediatrics, Delhi 1988.
14. Wahidan MH, Serie C, Germanier R, et al: A controlled field trial of live oral typhoid vaccine Ty21a. Bull WHO 1980, 58:469.
15. Wahidan MH, Serie C, Carisier R et al. A controlled field trial of live *salmonella typhi* strain Ty 21 a oral vaccine against typhoid: Three year results. J Infec Dis 1982, 145:292-295.

CHOLERA VACCINE

1. **Contents:** (i) 6000 million killed bacteria of Ogawa serotype of classical vibrio cholerae.
   (ii) 6000 million killed bacteria of Inaba serotype of classical vibrio cholerae.
2. **Ideal Age of primary vaccination:** Not recommended.
3. **Schedule of Primary vaccination :** Not applicable.
4. **Boosters:** Not applicable.
5. **When recommended:**
   - Previously recommended for international travel, now not required (W.H.O.)
   - Not useful in epidemics.
6. **Dose:** 0.25ml in <10 years.
   0.5 ml in >10 years.
   2 doses at 2-4 weeks interval.
7. **Route of administration :** Subcutaneous.
8. **Site of administration:**
   Deltoid or anterolateral aspect of thigh.
9. **Preparation of site of administration:**
   Clean with antiseptic (spirit).
10. **Instructions to the mother after vaccination:**
    Give antipyretics in case of fever.
11. **Protection/efficacy:** 35-50% (for 3 months)
12. **Contra-indications :** None
13. **Side effects:** Fever & local pain.
14. **Complications :** None.
15. **Storage at different levels and at doctor's clinic:**
    a) **When the vaccine is not is use :**
    In lowermost compartment of fridge (Do Not Freeze)
    b) **During immunization session.**
    Can be kept at room temperature.
    c) **In case of electricity failure:** Keep at cool & dark place.

NB : Presently available cholera vaccine is not useful for clinical purposes.

CHOLERA VACCINE 8

Dr. Raju Shah (RS) & Dr. Vijay Agarwal (VA)

Q.1. What is the dosage schedule of cholera vaccine and what are its side effects?

The schedule is mentioned in Table 1

Table 1
Recommended schedule of Cholera Vaccine

Age	*1st dose*	*2nd dose*
1-10 yrs	0.25 ml	0.25 ml
> 10 yrs	0.5 ml	0.5 ml

Side effects and complications are :

i. Abscess formation.

ii. Fever.

iii. Pain and restriction of movement of limbs.

iv. Rarely anaphylaxis.

Q.2. Cholera Vaccine is given by different authorities in case of epidemic situation. Is it a correct practice? Or should we immunize the children before epidemic.

No, it is not proper to give cholera vaccination during epidemic situations. It only creates a false sense of security. It has no effect on disease transmission. It is far better to concentrate on sanitation and water supply. It has no role in prevention of epidemics.

Q.3. Cholera vaccine administration is prerequisite for joining religious congregations. Is this a right practice ?

No. This is no more required even in our country.

Q.4. Some good schools demand cholera vaccination certificate, Why ?

This is due to old traditions and prejudices. Correct information is not supplied to them. They are further misled by misuse of cholera vaccine during epidemics by the authorities.

Q.5. Some countries still demand cholera vaccination while other have stopped demanding such certificates. What is the basis of this?

Now, that it is known that cholera vaccine is not a very useful vaccine, most countries do not demand this certificate. WHO has removed this vaccine from international heath regulations since 1973. However a valid certificated of cholera vaccine within preceding 6 months, is still required by some Middle-east countries in the mistaken belief that it is still effective.

Q.6. How can the household contacts of cholera be protected ?

The best way to protect household contacts of cholera is by ensuring high standards of sanitation and hygiene and by giving boiled and cooled water for drinking.

Some authorities suggest chemoprophylaxis with tetracyclines for household contacts. Dose recommended is 500mg B.D. for 2 days for adults.

Q.7. What are your comments on the efficacy of presently available cholera vaccine ?

It is a useless vaccine. Its efficacy is less than 50% and that too for 3 months or so.

Q.8. Are there any vaccines in the making which may be more effective in preventing cholera.

Two types of cholera vaccines are in various stages of development and may be more effective than the presently available one. These are :

a) Killed oral cholera vaccine, and

b) Lived attenuated oral vaccine. This appears to be more promising. A live attenuated oral vaccine (Texas star-SR), has shown antibodies in 93% recipients.

Q.9. Do you use cholera vaccine in your practice ?

As already stated, the presently available cholera vaccine is not at all effective, while it produces quite a few side effects. Hence this vaccine is useless and none of us use it in our practice.

Bibliography

1. Levin MM. Black RE Clements ML et al: Present status of cholera vaccines: Biochem. Soc Trans. 1984. 12:200-2.
2. Merson M H. Cholera. In Nelson's Text Book of Pediatrics Ed. RE Behrman and VC Vaughan, W.B. Saunders & Co., Philadelphia, 13th Edition pp 607.
3. Prasad VK and Kumar H. Cholera. In Immunisation practices in children. Ed. A.K. Dutta, S.K. Mittal and V. Agarwal. Indian Academy of Pediatrics, Delhi 1988.
4. WHO Memoranda. Recent advances in cholera research. Bull WHO 1985, 63: 841-9.

HEPATITIS B VACCINE

1. **Contents:** i) Plasma derived vaccine (Alum adsorbed)
   -20 ucg/ml (Hoechst)
   -5 ucg/ml (Curewell India)
   ii) Recombinant DNA Vaccine (20 µ cg/ml) SKF
2. **Ideal age for primary vaccination :** Not indicated
3. **Schedule of primary vaccination :** Not indicated
4. **Boosters :** Not indicated
5. **Dose :** 0.5 - 1 ml
   a) Schedule for pre-exposure prophylaxis
   1 ml at 0,1 and 6 months. Double the dose in patients on hemodialysis and immuno-compromised hosts.
   b) In Post exposure prophylaxis
   Perinatal 0.5 ml I.M. at 0-7 D, 1 month and 6 months (3 Doses)
   HBIG: One dose 0.5 ml at birth (<12 hrs).
   Accidental Exposure
   (Blood, Percutaneous): 1ml 0-7 D, 1 months & 6 months (3 doses)
   HBIG: 0.06 ml/kg (max.5 ml) immediately after exposure (<24 hrs.).
6. **Route of administration :** Intramuscular.
7. **Site of administration :**
   Deltoid (upper arm)/anterolateral aspect of thigh.
8. **Preparation of site for administration :**
   Clean with antiseptic (spirit).
9. **Instruction to the mother after vaccination:** None.
10. **Protection/Efficacy:** 95%
11. **Contra-indication:** None, (can be used in pregnancy also if required).
12. **Side effects:** Pain & erythema at local site.
13. **Complications :** None.
14. **Storage at different levels and at doctor's clinic:**
   a) **When the vaccine is not in use:**
   At+2° C to + 8° C in uppermost compartment of fridge.
   d) **During immunisation session :** Not applicable.
   c) **In case of electricity failure :** Ice box.

HEPATITIS B VACCINE 9

Dr. (Mrs) A.B. Desai (ABD) & Dr. AT Parathasarthy (ATP)

Q.1. What is the incidence of hepatitis B infection? Is it more than hepatitis A or non A non B hepatits?

Epidemiology of hepatitis infection is different in different part of the world. The incidence of hepatitis of different types varies according to the type of situations and according to age. Sporadic hepatitis in children in our country is more often due to hepatitis A while almost all the known epidemics in India have been due to non A non B hepatitis.

Table 1 shows the incidence in different situations, as reported in India. Table II gives the incidence in various groups of individuals.

Table I

Incidence of Various Hepatitis in Different Groups of Individuals.

	H.A.V.	H.B.V.	N.A.N.B.
Medical personnel	-	80	20
Male homosexuals	35	60	5
Drug addicts	20	60	20
Travellers	80	15	5

Table II

Incidence of Various Types of Hepatitis Agents In India.

	Sporadic Hepatitis		*Fulminant Hepatitis*	*Subacute Hepatitis*	*Post trans-fusion Hepatitis*
	Adult %	*Children* %	%	%	%
HAV	14	67	12	6	0
HBV	42	9	36	48	5
NANB	44	24	52	46	95

Different countries of world have been classified as per the prevalence of Hepatitis B infection. (Table III). Most of the countries of the West, fall in the low endemicity areas while countries of the South East Area like Thailand, Korea, Taiwan etc. fall in the high endemicity areas. India falls in the intermediate endemicity area with a carrier prevalence rate of 2.5-4.0% of HBV. Higher rates of HBV infection are also found in some parts of the country esp in South India.

Table III
Endemicity of Hepatitis B

Area	Carriers	Signs of Previous Infection
Low endemicity	Less than 2%	Less than 20%
Intermediate endemicity	2-7%	20-55%
High Endemicity	more than 7%	more than 55%

Q.2. Recently there is lot of mention of various markers of hepatitis infection in different text books. Is it necessary for a practising doctor to know about these markers. If so what is their utility in clinical practice ?

Viral hepatitis is caused by a variety of viruses namely hepatitis A (HAV), hepatitis B (HBV) and non A non B (NANB) viruses. Epidemiology of these three infections including their mode of spread, methods of prevention and their effects on the host differ from each other. It is important to understand these viruses and their various sero markers (antigens, antibodies to various components of these viruses) to be able to give rational advice to the patient regarding prevention and management of the concerned infection.

Hepatitis A virus (HAV) : This causes short incubation illness which spreads by orofecal route. This virus is excreted for a very brief period in the stool prior to onset of jaundice and the viremia with HAV is even more transitory, so hepatitis A antigen is not detectable in the blood. The more relevant index of infection with hepatitis A is the detection of IgM type of antibodies against hepatitis A virus which appear two to three weeks after infection and are detectable in the blood till 3 months after the infection. Thus presence of HAV IgM is the only seromarker which can help in diagnosing recent hepatitis A infection. There is no carrier state described with hepatitis A infection. The presence of HAV IgG antibodies in the serum suggests an old infection and an immunity to further infection to HAV.

Hepatitis B (HBV) : Hepatitis B or long incubation hepatitis is spread by the parenteral route and has a comparatively longer period of viremia making it possible to detect the antigen in the serum of the infected individuals.

Hepatitis B virus is a complex virus consisting of a number of antigens (Fig 1) each of which induces the production of type specific antibodies in the blood of infected individuals.

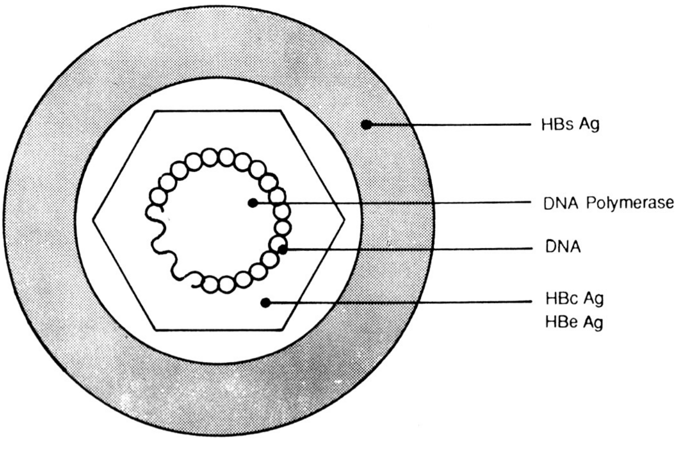

Fig. 1 Antigens of Hepatitis B virus

HBsAg is the best known antigen of the HBV and is its surface antigen (HBsAg, Australia antigen) which may be detectable in the blood for varying periods of time. HBV is known to produce a carrier state which is characterised by HBsAg in the blood for more than 6 months. The presence of antibodies against HBsAg (HBsAb) is suggestive of an old infection and protection against HBV infection. Inability to produce these antibodies may be responsible for development of carrier state.

HBcAg is the core antigen of HBV which is detectable only in the liver tissue. This antigen is not detectable in the blood. However IgM type of antibodies (HBcIgM) against this antigen are first to appear in the blood following HBV infection and hence are an indicator of recent HBV infection.

HBeAg is another core antigen of the hepatitis B virus which causes antigenemia. Presence of HBeAg in the blood indicates infectivity of the individuals and it is estimated that more than 90% individuals who carry HBeAg in the blood will transmit infection to others. The presence of antibodies against HBeAg suggests that the person is unlikely to transmit infection.

Non A Non B virus : This type of hepatitis virus infection is associated with both orofecal and parenteral route of spread. While in tropical countries, orofecal route seems to be more important, resulting in epidemics; in the temperate climates the parenteral route of spread appears to be more common. There are no known markers of this infection and diagnosis depends on excluding hepatitis A and hepatitis B infection.

Delta virus : This is a recently described hepatitis virus believed to be responsible for episodes of fulminant hepatitis occuring in hepatitis B carrier individuals. Its epidemiology in our country is not known.

In Western countries, non A non B virus infection was associated with parenteral route of spread. Recently a new virus particle named as Hepatitis C (HCV) has been isolated in these cases. It is now believed that Hepatitis C is responsible for almost 90% of transfusion associated hapatitis not due to Hepatitis B. Methods have also become available to detect antibodies to HCV by ELISA technique which can be used to screen potential blood donors.

On the other hand in developing countries like ours, the spread of Non A non B virus is associated predominantly with an oro-fecal route of spread and it is believed that a different viral particle (tentatively named as Hepatitis E) is responsible for this type of non A non B hapatitis. No specific markers are however as yet available for Hepatitis E.

Q.3. What is the usual clinical course of Hepatitis B infection.

In general the clinical picture resembles that of hepatitis A or non-A, non-B infection, but tends to be more severe.

In many patients the disease is not accompanied by jaundice and is termed anicteric, while a minority develop significant jaundice (icteric infection). In a few patients the disease follows an exceptionally severe course, known as fulminant hepatitis, which is often fatal. In these cases co-occurrence of delta infection has generally been reported. Most patients recover uneventfully, but in a small proportion the virus is not eliminated and a carrier state is established.

Q.4. What is the risk of becoming a carrier after HBV infection ?

In low endemicity areas most cases of acute infection are followed by full recovery, with the appearance of protective anti-HBs antibodies and the clearance of the virus form the body. In a small proportion of infection in adolescents and adults (about 5-10%), the virus is not cleared form the body as characterized by the presence of hepatitis B surface antigen (HBsAg) in repeat blood specimens for more than 6 months. The carrier state is much more likely to follow a non-icteric infection than an icteric one. Also males are much more likely to become carriers than females. Also carrier rates are higher if infection is acquired at a younger age.

In areas of high endemicity, infection occurs at a very young age, Indeed, infants born to carrier mothers usually acquire the infection at or soon after birth. They rarely suffer clinical illness, but are at very high risk of becoming carriers (90%).

A carrier state is defined only when the HBsAg persist in blood for more than 6 months.

Q.5. What is the risk of hepatocellular carcinoma in a carrier ?

There is a strong epidemiological association between markers of HBV infection and primary hepatocellular carcinoma (PHC). Up to 80% of cases of liver cancer in Asia have been attributed to hepatitis B infection. In the USA, it has been estimated that the risk of developing primary hepatocellular carcinoma is 12-300 times greater in carriers than in non-carriers.

There is probably a high correlation between infection early in life and the incidence of liver cancer.

Q.6. Which tests are employed to screen blood donors for Australia antigen? How reliable are these tests ?

ABD : Two assay methods are available. They are sufficiently sensitive for routine use and have equivalent sensitivity.

1. Radioimmune assay (RIA)
2. Enzyme linked immunoassay (ELISA)

The RIA agents are less stable and entail a far greater burden on the environment, so at present the ELISA is preferred.

ATP : Care must be taken to exclude false positive and false negative tests by repeating the test and by obtaining other sero markers.

Reverse Hemagglutidin assay (RPHA) is also very reliable and can even give the titres of Australia antigen in the serum, which are correlated with the infectivity of the individual. Studies in Taiwan have shown that a RPHA titre in pregnant mothers, of > 2550 HBs Ag are associated with increased risk of perinatal transmission of hepatitis B infection.

Q.7. Blood banks refuse to take blood if there is a history of jaundice in the donor. Does it mean that all cases of jaundice are due to Hepatitis B. Can other types of jaundice like HAV or Non A Non B hepatitis be transmitted through blood transfusion?

Not all cases of jaundice are due to Hepatitis B. But as stated earlier, NANB infection can also be transmitted through the parenteral route. This is fairly common infection in our country and there is no way to detect the presence (or infectivity) of this infection in the blood. It is for this reason that blood banks refuse to take blood from individuals who give history of jaundice in the past. HAV is not transmitted through blood.

Recently technique for diagnosing HCV infection has become available and should be utilised to screen blood donors and also to understand the epidemiology of this disease in our country.

Q.8. Is it not advisable to screen all patients of jaundice for the type of hapatitis especially Hepatitis B. What are the minimum tests which can be done to identify the type of jaundice? Where are these tests done?

Yes, it will be desirable to screen all cases of jaundice if facilities exist. Hepatitis B infection can be diagnosed by presence of HBsAg and by anti HBc IgM antibodies (not routinely available). Australia antigen is done in almost all big cities. Hepatitis A infection is diagnosed by showing HAVIgM antibodies (again not routinely available). There is no known method to positively diagnose NANB hepatitis (except HCV) and it remains a diagnosis of exclusion.

Even if, other tests are not available at least HBsAg should be asked for in all the cases of jaundice. Patients who are positive for HBsAg should be followed for development of carrier state. Intrepretation of different markers is given in Table IV.

Table IV
Differential diagnosis of viral hepatitis

Marker	Interpretation
IgM anti-HAV+	recent hepatitis A infection
IgM anti-HAV–/ IgG anti-HAV+	past hepatitis A infection
HBsAg+/HBeAg+ IgM anti-HBc+	recent hepatitis B infection
HBsAg+ (more than 6 months)	establishment of a carrier state.
HBsAg+/HBeAg+	high infectivity of the patient
Anti-HBe+	low infectivity of the patient
anti-HBs+	immunity to HBV (disease or vaccine induced)
Liver enzyme increase/other virus markers- for recent infection	non-A, non-B, hepatitis*
HBsAg+/Delta+/ anti-Delta+	superinfection or co-infection with the delta agent

* Test for HCV antibodies to detect HCV infection.

Q.9. Should we not screen all pregnant mothers for hepatitis B carrier state during antenatal check-up?

ABD : It may be desirable to screen all pregnant women, but it is not feasible to do it in all places. For HB virus carriers; status of HBeAg marker is the important one as it is more indicative of infectivity and this is not performed in most places. Routine screening may be desirable in countries like Taiwan, Korea, China, Japan where there are very high carrier rates (5 to 30%) but in India where carrier rate is only 2-7% and HBeAg positivity rate of less than 20% (among HBsAg positive individuals), this routine screening cannot be recommended. In India even today less than 50% women receive routine antenatal check-up. Considering the present status where even hemoglobin estimation and blood group of all antenatal women is not done, it is far fetched to recommend routine screening for HBs and HBe.

ATP: The following high risk women are recommended for prenatal HBsAg screening:

i) Acute or chronic live disease/or jaundice in the past.
ii) Working or having received treatment in a hemodialysis unit.
iii) Working or residing in an institution for the mentally retarded.
iv) Rejection as a blood donor.
v) Blood transfusion on repeated occasions.
vi) Frequent occupational exposure to blood in medical-dental settings.
vii) Household contact with an HBV carrier or hemodialysis patient.
viii) Multiple episodes of venereal diseases.
ix) Percutaneous use of illicit drugs.

Q.10. Do all Australia antigen positive mothers transmit hepatitis B infection to the newborn? If not how can we predict perinatal transmission?

Perinatal transmission can occur when mothers are HBsAg positive particularly when they are also HBeAg positive. On the other hand HBsAg positive, but HBeAg negative mothers are not totally free from HBV transmission but the risk of infection is considerably lower (<10%) in them (Table V) Similarly the infants of HBeAg positive nursing mothers are also at high risk.

Table V
Vertical transmission of HBV

Carrier state of the mother	Probability of infection of the newborn
HBsAg+/HBeAg+	65-90%
HBsAg+/HBeAg–	5-30%

Lowest incidence of the infection is seen when the mother has anti HBeAg antibodies

Q.11. If an infant is born to Australia antigen positive mother, how should the baby be protected.

HBIG in the dose of 0.5 ml IM should be given as part of neonatal care as soon as possible, in any case within 12 hours of birth, followed by HB vaccine 0.5 ml (10 microgram) IM within 7 days and repeated at 1 and 6 months of age. Another schedule which has been recommended is of giving HBV at 0, 1 and 2 month of age. This schedule ensures adequate antibodies by 3 months of age but a decline may occur is some children neccessiating a booster at 12 months of age.

As pointed above, not all HBsAg positive mothers transmit hepatitis to new borns. It would be preferable to obtain HBeAg also of the mother and to restrict hepatitis

B prophylaxis only to off springs of HBeAg positive mothers.

Infection to the newborn occurs at or around the time of birth. Hence immediate action starting in the new born period can prevent neonatal infection.

Q.12. There are two types of HB vaccines available viz. Plasma dervied and recombinant DNA vaccine. Which one is better?

Both are equally efficacious, but recombinant DNA (R-DNA) vaccine is better because of many reasons.

i) The cost of R-DNA is going to be much less, as it can be produced on a mass scale. This vaccine also has batch to batch consistency, high purity and immunogenicity

ii) Plasma derived vaccine has the potential risk of transmitting infection like AIDS or other (as yet unknown) infections.

Q.13. A person has accidentally received Australia antigen positive blood. What should be done ?

HBIG 0.06 ml/kg (maximum 5 ml) within 12-24 hours of transfusion followed by 3 doses of HB vaccine (20 µgm each dose) given at 0-7 days, 1 month and 6 months, will protect the recipient.

HBV should be given even if HBIG is not available.

Q.14. I have drawn blood sample of an Australia antigen positive patient. I was not wearing gloves at the time of taking blood sample. I do not have injuries or scratches on my hand. Should I still take HB vaccine or HBIG.

Medical professional and paramedical personnels working in laboratories are always at risk and ideally should receive pre-exposure prophylactic vaccinations (3 doses) against hepatitis B infection. However if this has not been done, then an exposure like the one described, should warrant immediate prophylaxis as outlined in the previous question. Absence of visible scratches is no guarantee that the infection cannot spread, as minor, non visible abrasions are sufficient to allow the entry of the virus into the body.

Q.15. A person has suffered from jaundice 5 years ago. Does he need hepatitis B vaccine now ?

Jaundice could have been due to any one of the hepatitis virus. Now his HBs Ag and anti HBsAb status should be studied. If they are both negative then he is still susceptible and may be given the vaccine (if he is at high risk).

Q.16. Should Australia antigen positive patients be given hepatitis B vaccine?

As the infection has already occured there is no need for the vaccine.

Q.17. Is the efficacy of HB vaccine same in immunocompromised individuals as in normal ones ?

Seroconversion rates with standard dose (20 µg each x 3) is about 60-70% in immuno-compromised individuals and in patients on hemodialysis. It has been suggested to either give 3 doses of 40 µg each to these individuals or to give one additional dose of HBV after 2 months of the of third dose to ensure protection. If available, antibody levels should be obtained in all these individuals.

Q.18. Can HB vaccine be used for pre-exposure prophylaxis ? if so who should receive it, what schedule should be followed ?

Yes, it can be used for pre-exposure prophylaxis.
Following categories of personnel should receive pre-exposure prophylaxis:

i) Health care personnels such as doctors, nurses, technicians, staff working in laboratories, blood banks, dialysis units, postmortem room.
ii) Recipients of blood and blood products such as patients in hematology-oncology units, those on dialysis, cases of thalassemia, sickle cell disease, leukemia, hemophilia, immunodeficiency diseases and malignancy.
iii) Personnel and residents of institutions like those for mentally handicapped, where prolonged institutionalisation is necessary.
iv) Household contacts and sexual partners of HBV carriers.
v) Illicit users of injectable drugs.
vi) International travellers to endemic areas.

Recommended schedule for pre-exposure prophylaxis is :

3 doses of Hepatitis B vaccine (20ug each) given at 0, 1 and 6 months. It can also be given at 0, 1 & 2 months if quicker response is required but then a booster should also be given at 12 months.

NB : i) Vaccine should be given over deltoid region.
ii) Dose is same for both children and adults.
iii) For patients on hemodialysis and those immunocompromised, additional dose is given 2 months after the 3rd dose.

Q.19. What is the current recommendations for HB vaccine booster ?

If a schedule of 0, 1 and 6 months has been adopted a booster dose is recommended after 5 years. On the other hand if the vaccine has been given according to 0, 1 and 2 month schedule, a booster should be given at 12 months. This will ensure adequate protection for about 8 years.

If facility for anti HBs antibody determination is available, then a booster should be administered only when this antibody level has fallen below 10 I.U./L. It will be more important to ensure this, in patients who are likely to respond poorly to the vaccine (such as immunocompromised and hemo dialysed patients).

Q.20. What is the role of HBIG in the prevention of hepatitis B infection?

The role of HBIG is limited to post exposure situations only. Its usefulness is well documented in perinatal, percutaneous and sexual post exposure situations. HBIG given alone twice one months apart gives 75% protection but it should always be followed by active immunisation with hepatitis B vaccine.

Q.21. Can HBIG and HB vaccine be given concurrently? Which are the conditions when both are given simultaneously?

Yes, HBIG and HB vaccine can be given simultaneously as HBIG does not interfere with simultaneous hepatitis B vaccine. This is most useful in newborn babies of HBe positive mothers and in postexposure prophylaxis, HBIG and hepatitis B vaccine should be given by different syringes at different sites.

Q.22. Generally it is said that specific immunoglobulins and live viral vaccine should not be given simultaneously (e.g. measles vaccine and immunoglobulin) why then can the HBIG and HB vaccine be given together?

Good levels of protection are achieved even when HBIG and HB vaccine are given simultaneously. Protection with combined use is 90% while with HBIG alone it is only 75%. This is probably due to high potency of hepatitis B vaccine.

Q.23. Can HB vaccine and HBIG be combined in the same syringe and injected at the same site ?

No. They cannot be combined or injected at the same site. Separate syringes and separate sites are to be used.

Q.24. How should household contacts of a hepatitis B patient be protected.

They should be treated as high risk individuals. If they are not already immune, then they should also receive HBIG and prophylaxis with 3 doses of hepatitis B vaccine.

Q.25. Can the patient with hapatitis B carrier state be treated with HBIG?

It is of no value.

Q.26. Can Australia antigen positive mother breast feed her infant?

Yes breast feeding can be given.

Q.27. How should HB vaccine be stored.

The vaccine should be stored at 2° to 8°C. It should never be frozen.

Q.28. What is the efficacy of HB vaccine ?

The efficacy is excellent. Specific antibodies appear in 95-100% of vaccinees who receive 3 doses.

Q.29. What are the contraindications ?

There are no specific contraindications. It can be used even in pregnancy. Non specific contraindications include severe febrile conditions and known hypersensitivity to any components of the vaccine.

Q.30. A person has been exposed to HB infection. He cannot afford HBIG. Should he still be given the vaccine ?

It is true that many patients cannot afford HBIG as one ampoule of it costs about seven thousand rupees. In any case even if HBIG cannot be given, HB vaccine should be given in complete (0, 1, 2 & 12 months) schedule. This will ensure early and sustained protection, although less than the combined use of HBIG & HB vaccine.

It has been shown clearly in newborns that HB vaccine alone is protective in more than 90% patients.

Q.31. A person has received 3 doses of plasma derived vaccine. Can he now receive DNA recombinant vaccine for booster ?

Yes, it is possible to shift to DNA vaccine at any stage in the vaccination course. The antibody response to DNA vaccine is qualitatively and quantitatively similar to that from plasma derived vaccine.

Q.32. Can healthy pregnant or nursing mother be given hepatitis B vaccine ?

Vaccination during pregnancy is not generally recommended. However if a high risk situation exists, then active immunisation with HB vaccine can be undertaken even in pregnant women.

There is no reason why lactating mothers cannot be given HB vaccine.

Q.33. Can Hepatitis B vaccine be given with other vaccine ?

Yes, hapatitis B vaccine can be given with most of the EPI vaccines, except measles (or MMR) vaccine which may be theoritically contraindicated (because of possible immunosuppressive role of measles vaccine).

Q.34. Can recipients of R-DNA vaccine be accepted as blood donors ?

Recipients receive surface antigen and not the whole virus particle and hence cannot transmit infection. Further vaccinees develop anti HBs antibodies which are protective to the individual.

Bibliography

1. American Academy of Pediatrics, 1986. Report of the Committee of Infectious Diseases.
2. Balistreri WF, Viral hepatitis PCNA. 1988, 35: 637-669.
3. Dienstay JL, Wards JR and Koh RS: Acute hepatitis. In: Harrison's Principles of Internal Medicine. Editors: Peterdorf, Adams and Braunwald et al. 10th Edition, 1983, pp 1789-1794.
4. Edwards MS. Hepatitis B serology, help in interpretations P.C.N.A. 1988, 35: 503-515.
5. Madhulika S, Kumar H: Viral hepatitis: In Immunization Practices in Children. Editied by A Dutta et al Indian Academy of Pediatrics Delhi 1988 page 75-82.
6. Okada K. Kamiyama I, Inomata Metal. Antigen e and anti e in the serum of asymptomatic carrier mothers as indicators of passive and negative transmission of HBV to their infants. NEJM 1976, 294: 746-49.
7. Pontecarvo, M: Vaccines, sera, immunolobulin: Practical Hand book 1985. Minerva Medical Publishers, 1985. pp 26-27.
8. Sleveus CE, Neurath RA, Besley RP et al. HbeAg and ante HBe detection by radio-immunoassay: Correlation with vertical transmission of hepatitis B virus in Taiwan. J Med Viro 1979, 3: 237-42.
9. Stevens EC, Toy PT, Tong MJ et al. Perinatal hepatitis B virus transmission in the United States. Prevention by passive-active immunization. JAMA 1985, 253: 1740-1744.
10. Tandon BN, Gandhi BM and Joshi YK. Etiological specturm of viral hepatitis and prevalence of markers of hepatitis A & B virus infection in North India. WHO Bulletin 1984 62: 67-73.

RABIES : TISSUE CULTURE VACCINE

1. **Contents:**
   a) HDCV (Human Diploid Cell Vaccine) : Contains rabies virus (Wister rabies PMW1 38-1503-3M strain) obtained from culture on human diploid cells, inactivated by beta-propiolactone (2.5 IU)
   b) PCEC : Rabies virus grown on purified chick embryo cells, inactivated by beta-propiolactone.
2. **Ideal age of Primary vaccination:** Not recommended
3. **Schedule of Primary vaccination** : Not recommended
4. **Boosters:** Not applicable
5. **When recommended:**
   (i) Pre-exposure prophylaxis (to high risk) D0, D7 & D28
   (ii) post exposure prophylaxis D0, D3, D7, D14, D28, D90
6. **Dose:** 1 ml each
7. **Route of administration** : IM (PCEC), SC/IM (HDCV)
8. **Site of administration:** Deltoid region.
9. **Preparation of site of administration:**
   Clean with antiseptic (spirit).
10. **Instructions to the mother after vaccination:** None
11. **Protection/efficacy:** Almost 100%.
12. **Contra-indications** :
    Nil (Possibility of rabies overrides any other consideration).
13. **Side effects:** Nil
14. **Complications** : Nil
15. **Storage at different levels and at doctor's clinic:**
    a) **When the vaccine is not is use** :
       2° - 8° C in upper compartment of fridge.
    b) **During immunization session** : Not applicable.
    c) **In case of electricity failure:** Ice box.

RABIES VACCINE

Dr. R.K. Puri (RKP)

Q.1. Which animal bites can be rabid? Can rat bite cause rabies ?

Bites by rabid dog, cat, fox or bat can cause rabies. Rat bites usually do not cause rabies in humans as they are less commonly infected.

Monkey bites and rat bites are extremly rare cause of rabies but nevertheles, rabies prophylaxis would be indicated even in these cases. Cattles are well known sources of rabies to man. Among the wild animals mongoose, racoons etc. can also harbour rabies virus. In India 96% of rabies is caused by dog bites.

Q.2. Is man to man transmission of rabies possible?

Man to man transmission is virtually not reported. However transmission of rabies by corneal transplant from patient with undiagnosed rabies encephalitis, to healthy recipients has been reported.

Individuals attending to hydrophobia patients should take all precautions to ensure that they are not accidently bitten by the patient. Saliva of the patient should also not come in contact with any fresh cut or abrasion on the skin or the mucous membranes in their body. If any attendent has handled excretion/secretion of a case of hydrophobia he must be given complete anti-rabies prophylaxis.

Q.3. Is mere contact with a rabid animal or patient sufficient enough to cause rabies?

No. But if the saliva of a rabid animal or patient comes in contact with broken skin or mucous membrane, rabies can occur in the contacts.

Q.4. Is oral transmission of rabies virus possible, for instance through ingestion of milk?

Oral transmission is not possible as the virus is destroyed in the stomach. However, if oral ulcers are present, transmission may occur in 20% of cases particularly if the milk is ingested without boiling.

Q.5. What about transplacental transmission of rabies ?

As rabies virus is of high molecular weight, it cannot be transported across the placental barrier.

Q.6. Should antirabies vaccine be a part of the immunization schedule of children as most of the children love to play with dogs ?

No. As every dog is not rabid, it is not necessary to include this vaccine in the immunization schedule.

Children love to play with dogs and not necessarily pet dogs alone. Some authorities have recommended including children among the list of high risk individuals who may be considered for pre-exposure prophylaxis. It is however not cost effective to be included in the routine immunisation schedules. It must be remembered that only tissue culture vaccines like human diploid cell vaccine (HDCV) or purified chick embryo cell (PCEC) can be used for pre-exposure prophylaxis.

Boosters of Rabies Vaccine can lead to hypersensitivity reactions and hence routine prophylaxis should not be used indiscriminatily.

Q.7. Hydrophobia-the hallmark of diagnosis of rabies is present in just 50 percent of cases. The remaining cases (eg presenting as encephalities) may be unknowingly handled by doctors. Do you recommend routine vaccination of doctors against rabies ?

Yes. All doctors who treat rabies actively and those who undertake corneal grafting, should receive pre-exposure prophylaxis.

At times patients with rabies are admitted with presentations simulating encephlitis, meningitis, poliomyelitis or other paralytic illnesses. These pose special dangers to the attending staff as they often fail to take neccessary precautions to avoid exposure. Therefore it is recommended that all medical and paramedical personnel who are likely to come in contact with a rabies case, should receive pre-exposure prophylaxis.

Q.8. Who else should receive pre-exposure prophylaxsis ?

Laboratory staff, veterinary surgeons, wild game wardens in endozootic areas, naturalists, forestry workers, taxidermists and country postmen should receive pre-exposure prophylaxis.

Morning walkers have also been included in the list by some authorities.

Whenever you have to decide about pre exposue prophylaxis, the relative risk of contacting rabies versus the risk from hypersensitivity reaction due to boosters of rabies vaccine, should be carefully weighed. People who have a low risk of rabies face a greater danger from hypersensitive reaction to rabies boosters.

Q.9. What is the schedule of pre-exposure Immunization ?

WHO recommends 3 dose schedule on 0, 7 and 28 days or 0, 28 and 56 days.

Only tissue culture vaccines (PCEC or HDCV should be used for pre-exposure prophylaxis.

Q.10. What are the advantages of pre-exposure vaccination?

Advantages of pre-exposure prophylaxis are :

i) It creates basic immunity which will be of great value in event of contact with rabid animal.

ii) It limits the risk caused by delays necessary to obtain vaccine.

iii) It renders the injection of antirabies immunoglobulin unnecessary.

iv) It reduces the number of vaccine doses in post exposure treatment.

Q.11. HDCV is preferred to be given through subcutaneous route while PCEC is given through intramuscular route. Why is there a difference in the route of aminlstration?

Different route are preferred because of differences in moleculer weight and the level of dispersion of the two vaccines. PCEC if given subcutaneously is known to produce local necrosis and/or abscess because of its high molecular weight.

Q.12. A child has been bitten by a dog, suspected to be rabid. How should the wound be managed? should it be cleaned with spirit or cauterized?

The wound should be throughly washed with soap and water. Cauterization should not be used. Stiching should also be postponed if possible.

Washing of the wound is most important. It should be done very thoroughly, even if the patient has reported days or weeks after the bite. Antiseptics are not much helpful. It is better to wash away the virus then to try and kill it with antiseptics of doubtful efficacy.

Local serotherapy with rabies immune globulin RIG should be considered in cases of severe bites. Cauterization causes necrosis and further facilitates the travel of the virus from the skin to the nerves. Stitching of wounds should also be avoided. Tetanus prophylaxis should be done as indicated (See Chapter on DPT)

Q.13. Can rables wounds be sutured and if yes under what conditions should it be done?

The would should not be sutured straight away. It should be done only after 24-28 hours (if totally unavoidable) to avoid diffusion of rabies virus to nerve fibres. Anti serum or specific human rabies immune globulin (HRIG) should be irrigated carefully in and around the wound.

Q.14. A child is bitten over legs by an untraceable stray dog. What should be the management?

It should be automatically considered rabid and post exposure treatment should be started immediately.

Q.15. If the biting stray dog is traceble, should the dog be first observed for 10 days and then the immunization against rabies be decided accordingly.

No. The post exposure treatment should be started immediately as the dog may be potentially rabid. However, if the dog does not die at the completion of 10 days of observation, further treatment with vaccine may be stopped.

Q.16. What is the principle behind this observation phase of 10 days?

Usually virus is found in the saliva of the dogs, 3-5 days before the onset of disease and the disease lasts in dogs for about 5-6 days and hence the observation for 10 days.

No case of rabies has been attributed to a dog or a cat that has remained healthy throughout the 10 days period of observation.

Q.17. My pet dog (Immunized against rabies) died of sudden unexplained death. What should be done to the dog and for the family contacts?

The body should be handled with great care, and whole body or head and neck should be sent to nearest rabies diagnostic centre as soon as possible. The dog must be buried in 3-4 feet deep pit.

The family members should be started on post-exposure treatment till reports are available. If the report is negative, the treatment should be discontinued.

Q.18. Should postexposure vaccine be given to a person who has already taken pre-exposure prophylaxis.

Yes. he should have 3 doses of tissue culture vaccine on O, 3 & 7 days for full protection.

Same schedule can be followed if the person has received complete post exposure rabies vaccine treatment (with tissue culture vaccine) within the last 2 years. However, if more than 2 years has elapsed since the completion of pre/post exposure prophylaxis, then a complete course (of 6 doses) should be given.

Q.19. How does the management of cases differ in different types of animal bites viz. class I, Class II, & Class III ? Has the classification become obsolete after the advent of newer, effective and safer vaccines ?

The management is different in different types of animal bites when nerve tissue vaccine (NTV) is used. This is because the side effects of NTV are related to the dose of vaccine, and one likes to use the minimum amount of this vaccine, necessary to prevent rabies in different types of wounds. The classification has become obsolete after the advent of tissue culture vaccines because all individuals, whether bitten by suspected or definitely rabid animals must receive vaccine and the dose is the same irrespective of age or sex of the individual or the severity of bite. Safety of tissue culture vaccines has made the classification of wound unnecessary.

Q.20. Can neonates be given anti-rabies vaccine without any danger of side effects? Should the dose be reduced in newborns?

Yes, rabies vaccine can be given to new borns also. As the newborns are more susceptible to get severe disease after bite by rabid dog, they must receive same dose of HDCV. This vaccine does not produce any side effects. PCEC can also be used if HDCV is not available or cannot be afforded.

The dose of HDCV is same irrespective of age.

Q.21. Can children on steroids (or immunocompromised hosts) be given anti rabies vaccine?

All such individuals must get rabies vaccine because the danger of rabies far out weighes any possible risk with the vaccine. Antibody in serum must be tested to ensure that vaccination has been successful.

If possible immunosuppressive therapy (Steroids & other drugs) should be stopped during active immunisation with rabies.

Q.22. Can mealses vaccine be given to a child who is on post exposure prophylaxis?

It would be preferable to wait for at last 6 weeks after the last dose of rabies vaccine, before giving measles vaccination.

Q.23. A child has recently recovered from exanthema (Chicken-pox or Measles). Can this child be given rabies vaccine?

Yes, as risk of rabies overrides all other consideration. However seroconversion must be ensured.

Q.24. Can pregnant mother be administered anti-rabies vaccine?

Yes. Pregnancy does not constitute a contraindication to post exposure treatment if vaccination is important in any case of bites. In France, observation of twelve pregnant women on post exposure treatment did not show any adverse effects on fetus.

Q.25. Can lactating women be administered antirabies vaccine ?

Yes, it does not produce any harmful effects on infants.

Risk of rabies overrides all other consideration. Whenever in doubt, give rabies vaccine and if necessary check for adequate seroconversion.

Q.26. Which is the most appropriate site of antirabies vaccine? The manufacturer recommends deltoid region. In children can we give at sites other than deltoid region?

The ideal site of vaccination is deltoid region because this area is rich in lymphatics & is vascular. Vaccine efficacy is much better when used on deltoid region compared to any other site, and therefore deltoid area should be used.

Q.27. What are the indications of sero-therapy?

Immediate homologous serotherapy is a must in cases of any serious bite. Whether the animal is traceable or not, rabid or only suspected. Such bites include :–

i) Deep bites or scratches on face, head, neck, hands or feet.
ii) Multiple bites, wounds, scratches on body.
iii) Minor bites in neonates & young children
iv) Bites awaiting clinical confirmation

If Human Rabies Immune Globulin (HRIG) is available then all cases of bites by suspected rabid animal, must be given RIG as this provides immediate protection. Human rabies immune globulin is safe and hence can be easily used in all cases. However, if equine rabies immunoglobulin only is available then it may be advisable to restrict its use only in cases of severe bites, that too after skin testing. Serotherapy is not required if the person has already received pre-exposure prophylaxis.

Q.28. Can serotherapy be given after 48 hours of animal bites ?

Yes, serotherapy can be given upto 8 days after exposure or even later if active immunisation has not already been started. However it should be started as early as possible preferably in first 24 hours.

Q.29. Which is the most appropriate site for rabies immunoglobulin injection? How should it be administered, should it be sprayed or applied with swab or injected by multiple injections at bitten sites ?

Total dose of Human rabies immunoglobilin (HRIG) is 20 IU/kg. Half of this is given by intramuscular route either in the detoid region or on the lateral aspect of the thigh. The other half is used to irrigate the wound locally.

Dose of equine rabies immunoglobulin is 40 i.u./kg. Half of this is given intramuscular after skin testing and the other half is given around the wound. Spraying or applying with swab is not adequate.

Q.30. What could happen if immunoglobulin is not administered along with the vaccine in post-exposure prophylaxis?

After the first injection of HDC vaccine, immunity is acquired in about 7-10 days, and upto this time the child remains unprotected. The immunoglobulin provide immediate passive immunity to the subject and helps to ward off the development of active disease.

Normally rabies is a rather slow growing virus disease with a long incubation period which allows commencement of active immunization with the rabies vaccine after the person has been exposed to the virus. However, in certain cass the incubation period may be ultra short (even 5 days). Antibodies to rabies are induced only 7-10 days after the first dose of vaccine. RIG injected soon after exposure takes care during these 7-10 days by providing immediate passive immunity. Also RIG helps to prevent the migration of the virus along the neurones.

Q.31. Is the schedule for post exposure prophylaxis in persons same even if that person has received pre-exposure prophylaxis?

Only three doses of PCEC/HDCV are required in such cases on day 0, 3 & 7 (See Q 16). Serotherapy is not required in such cases.

Q.32. What are the advantages of tissue culture vaccines (PCEC/HDCV) over nerve tissue vaccine (NTV) ?

The advantages of tissue culture vaccines are :

i) Formation of high degree of neutralizing antibodies in a short period & hence a good immunogenecity. The efficacy of NTV is 50-60% while PCEC/HDCV vaccines are nearly 100% effective.

ii) Excellent local and general tolerance, hardly any side effects.

iii) No foreign virus or oncogenic nucleic acid.

iv) Small dose of 1 ml, given S/C or IM (same for all ages).

v) Total number of injections 5-6, spread over three months.

vi) Can be given as pre-exposure prophylaxis also.

Tissue culture vaccines are extremely safe. Side effects are uncommon and minor such as local pain, erythema, itching or mild systemic reactions. Rare cases of neuro-paralytic illness have also been reported following HDCV.

Q.33. What is the efficacy of NTV against rabies ? What about its side effects ?

Efficacy of NTV is variable and unpredictable. It has plenty of side effects which occurs in 20-25% of patients, some of them may even be fatal. Side effects increase with increasing number of doses and are :

a) *Local*: Moderate pain, redness, itching at the site of innoculation and rarely abscess.
b) *General*: Mild systemic reaction - fever, headache, giddiness, palpitation and diarrhea. Generalized urticaria, agioneurotic edema and shock may also occur.
c) *Neuroparalytic accidents*: These occur in 1 in 1100 to 1 in 800 treated cases as a result of sensitization of patients to sheep brain. Three types of neuropralytic attacks are seen viz. neuritic, lumbodorsal and Landry type.

Q.34. What is the justification for continued use of NTV vaccine in government hospitals and dispensaries ?

Justification for continued use of NTV in our government hospitals in the low cost of NTV. The total cost of treatment with NTV, HDC & PCEC vaccines is Rs. 30-40, 2500 and 1000/- respectively.

Despite apparently low cost, the continued use of NTV cannot be justified at all. If one is to calculate the cost, one must also include the cost of treatment failure (40-50% in NTV compared to nil with tissue culture vaccines) and the high incidence of neuroparalytic complications (1:1100 in N.T.V. vs almost nil in tissue culture vaccines). If the cost of all this is added, certainly tissue culture vaccine will turn out to be quite cost effective. If the government can spend crores of rupees on coronary care units, certainly it can afford better and safer vaccine against such a dreaded disease as rabies.

Q.35. Now that two types of tissue culture vaccines are available viz. HDCV and PCEC which is better and more effective ? Kindly tell us the schedule of administration of both vaccine.

The efficacy of both HDCV & PCEC vaccine is the same. Both vaccines provide almost 100% protection against rabies. Both are equally safe. The only difference being the 'cost' HDVC is three times costlier than PCEC. The dosage schedule for both vaccine is the same i.e. on day 0, 3, 7, 14, 30 and followed by one optional booster on the 90th day. The treatment must start as soon as possible. PCEC may provoke hypersensitive reactions in individuals allergic to egg.

Q.36. Intradermal injection of antirabies vaccine is recommended by an Indian Textbook of Pediatrics (by O.P. Ghai). Use of I.D. route will definetely save money. Are there sufficient studies available to justify this route of administration in prevention of such a dreadful disease?

Intradermal route has been advocated as its allows the use of only O.I ml per dose. This can be used for preexposure prophylaxis, under strict supervision and with demonstration of adequate antibody response after the completion of the course. At present it can not be recommended for postexposure prophylaxis as any vaccine failure would not be acceptable for such a dreaded disease as rabies. It must be cautioned that it is quite difficult to give intradermal injection and if the small dose meant for I.D. route has gone subcutaneous, it will be totally ineffective.

Q.37. Does the management of a provoked bite differ from an unprovoked bite ?

Children usually get bitten by their pet dogs as a result of undue provocation (like pulling the ears or the tails). These provoked bites by (presumably protected) pet dogs are normally harmless. On the other hand unprovoked bites even by pet dogs should be considered as bites by rabid animal. Provoked or unprovoked bites by stray animals should always be considered as possibly infectious.

Q.38. Can a vaccinated dog transmit rabies? How effective is dog vaccine?

Yes, even a vaccinated dog can transmit rabies especially if the dog has not received regular booster dose once in a year at proper times. The available dog vaccine (nerve tissue type), usually provides 65 to 70% immunity.

Q.39. Which is most effective dog vaccine? Please tell us its schedule also.

Live attenuated vaccine is said to be most effective vaccine for dogs. Other vaccines like (NTV & tissue culture) are also quite effective. However dogs under 3 months do not get immunized effectively. Schedule of live attenuated vaccine for dogs is as follows:

3 ml single dose followed by booster every 3 years.

Q.40. A child has been bitten by a 2 month old puppy? Should he also get anti rabies vaccine.

It is a difficult question to answer as there is no direct reference available for such a situation. However considering various facts, it is highly unlikely that the 2 month old puppy could be suffering from rabies because:

i) Transplacetal transfer of rabies virus is not known.

ii) Active immunisation of a puppy is not recommended before 3 months of age suggesting that the transplacentally transfered antibodies may be interfering with the development of immunity (however no direct reference is available for this).

Thus in all probability this child would not require any prophylaxis.

However in view of the possible doubt, this bite may be presumed to be to have been caused by a healthy pet and treated as such. Thus the puppy should be captured and observed for 10 days. If he develops any symptoms during this time he should be sacrificed and his brain examined for rabies virus. Rabies prophylaxis be started in the child as soon as the dog develops abnormal behaviour.

Q.41. A child has received three doses of tissue culture vaccine as a part of post exposure prophylaxis on day 0, 3, and 7. The dog is normal after 10 days. Should the further course of antirabies vaccination be stopped? In such a case are these three doses sufficient enough to be acknowledged as pre-exposure prophylaxis?

If the dog is normal after 10 days of observation, the vaccine can be stopped i.e. next dose need not be given. As these 3 doses are given on 0, 3, and 7 days, it can not be considered as pre-exposure prophylaxis because the schedule of prexposure prophylaxis is 0, 7 and 28 days. An additional dose on day 28 will ensure complete pre-exposure prophylaxis.

Q.42. A child has reported 10 days after a bite by an untracable dog, should this child be given antirabies vaccine or serum?

Yes, even if the child reports after 10 days, antirabies vaccine must be started along with one injection of rabies immunoglobulin.

Q.43. A child has received full course of post exposure antirabies prophylaxis one year ago. Once again he is bitten by a stray dog. Should the antirabies vaccine be given again? if yes then what should be the schedule?

For a subject in whom presence of antibodies had been demonstrated in the past, WHO Group recommends the injection of only one dose of HDCV vaccine on day 0. In subjects in whom antibody titers have not been checked, 3 doses should be given on day 0, 3 & 7.

As antibodies levels are usually not available, it will be preferable to give 3 doses of HDCV to all individuals re-exposed within 2 years.

Q.44. Does the schedule differ in case the bitten child was given full course of antirabies vaccine as a part of post-exposure prophylaxis 5 years back? Should antibody levels be done first to decide the schedule?

Antibodies decline in 2-3 years after a complete schedule of tissue culture vaccine. This child would therefore require a full course of vaccination.

Q.45. Can we take the same course of action if the child has been given NTV previously?

No, antibodies following NTV do not last more than 6 months. Hence these children would require a complete course of vaccination if they are exposed any time after 6 months of the initial treatment.

Q.46. A child has received first 3 doses of HDCV as a part of post exposure prophylaxis. Can the course be continued with PCEC, if HDCV is not available or patient is not able to afford HDCV?

Yes, if HDCV is not available, the course can be completed with PCEC because the extent of efficacy of both vaccines is the same, and basically both the vaccines contain the same virus.

Q.47. If by chance, a 4th or 5th dose of tissue culture vaccine is missed for some reason what should be further course of action? Should the schedule be started all over again?

If the 4th/5th dose of tissue culture vaccine is missed there is no need to restart the schedule because earlier doses have produced some immunity which has been registered in its immunological memory. Thus give 4th doses when the child is brought and give the further schedule accordingly.

Right at the initiation of the course, the parents must be warned that unless the whole course is taken at proper time, the treatment may not be effective. 4th and 5th dose (on day 14 & 28) produce a booster like action with brisk and marked antibody response. The virus usually reaches the target organ around this time and if adequate antibodies are not available then it will attach it self to the target organ. Once that happens, then no amount of antibody can affect the virus. Thus a timely administration of the vaccine (esp. its 4th & 5th dose) is most important. Nevertheless if the doses have been missed inadverantly, there in no need to restart the schedule.

Q.48. Does any drug interfere with development of adequate antibody response to antrabies vaccine?

It has been observed that chloroquine interferes in the development of adequate antibody response during pre-exposure prophylaxis. In the light of this observation it would be preferable to avoid chloroquin therapy during post-exposure treatment also.

Bibliography

1. Bernard KW, Smith PW, Kader FJ et al: Neuroparalytic illness and human diploid cell rabies vaccine JAMA 1982, 248: 3136.
2. Bijok U. Purified chick embryo cell (PCEC) rabies vaccine: a review of clinical development in: Improvement in Rabies post exposure treatment. (Eds: Vodopija I, Nicholson KG, Smerdel S and Bijok U) Zagreb Institute of Public health, Zagreb 1985, pp 103-111.
3. Centres for Disease Control: Systemic allergic reactions following immunization with human diploid cell rabies vaccines. MMWR 1984, 33:185.
4. Centres for Disease Control: Human rabies acquired outside the United States. MMWR 1985, 34:235.

5. Kumar H. and Prasad VK. Rabies. In Immunisation Practices in children. Ed. A Datta, SK Mittal and V Agarwal. Ind Acad of Pediatrics, Delhi, 1988.

6. Nicholson KG, Farrow PR, Bijok W, Barth R.: Pre-exposure studies with purified chick embryo cell culture rabies vaccine and human diploid cell vaccine: Serological and clinical responses in man. Vaccine 1987, 5, 208-210.

7. Pappioanu M, Fishbein DB, Dreesen DW et al. Antibody response to pre-exposure human diploid cell rabies vaccine given concurrently with chloroquine. N Engl J Med 1986, 314:280.

8. Rai chowdhuri AN, Bhatia, R: Ichupajani RL: Immunoprophylaxis against Rabies. J. Commun Dis 1984, 161(1) 43-48.

9. Sehgal, S, Bhatia R: Rabies-current status and proposed control programme in India. National Instt. of Communicable Diseases (Directorate General of Health Services), 1985.

10. Steinhoff MC, John TJ. Prevention and treatment of Rabies. Ind J Pediatr 1984, 51, 560-565.

11. Wiktor TJ. Peotkins S, Grella D.: Human cell culture rabies vaccine. JAMA 1973, 24: 1170-1171.

MENINGOCOCCAL VACCINE

1. **Contents:** Each unit dose contains purified lyophilised polysaccharide of *Neisseria meningitidis* Group A & C each 50ug.
2. **Ideal age of primary vaccination:** Not recommended
3. **Schedule of Primary vaccination :** Not recommended
4. **Boosters:** Not applicable
5. **When recommended:** During epidemics.
6. **Dose: 0.5 ml.**
7. **Route of administration :** Subscutaneous.
8. **Site of administration:**
   Upper arm/anterolateral aspect of thigh.
9. **Preparation of site of administration:**
   Clean with antiseptic (spirit).
10. **Instructions to the mother after vaccination:** Nil
11. **Protection/efficacy:** 90% (if used after the age of 2 years).
12. **Contra-indications :** None.
13. **Side effects:** Mild fever and local pain.
14. **Complications :** Nil
15. **Storage at different levels and at doctor's clinic:**
    a) **When the vaccine is not in use :**
       2° - 8° C in uppermost compartment of fridge.
    b) **During immunization session :**
       On ice, (use within 2 hours).
    c) **In case of electricity failure:** Keep in ice box.

MENINGOCOCCAL VACCINE 11

Dr. Arvind Taneja (AT) & Dr. A.T. Parthasarthy (ATP)

Q.1. Certain parts of our counrty have had meningitis (meningococcal) epidemic in recent past. Does it not warrant the use of meningitis vaccine routinely?

A Meningococcal epidemic occured in the years 1985, 1986 and 1987. At present sporadic cases are still occuring (endemic meningitis). But an epidemic is certainly not around and so the situation does not warrant the use of meningcoccal vaccine (A&C) routinely.

Epidemics are usually caused by group A strains and less often by group C strains and very rarely by group B strains (Brazil). Endemic meningococcal meningitis is usally caused by group B strain for which no effective vaccine is available.

Q.2. Can meningitis vaccine be given to prevent endemic form of meningitis ?

The incidence of endemic disease is so low that it is not cost effective to recommend its prevention by large scale vaccination.

As pointed above endemic form is mostly caused by Gr. B. meningococci against which no effective vaccine is available. Meningococcal vaccine presently available is effective against Gr. A & Gr. C meningococcus and hence cannot be used to prevent endemic form of disease.

Q.3. Manufacturers recommend that meningococcal vaccine to be given after the age of 2 years only. Why we can not use this vaccine before the age of 2 years ?

Meningococcal vaccine is actually the purified capsular polysaccharide (carbohydrate structure) antigen of Type

A & C strains (50 micrograms of each) The immune system of the human body usually does not respond well to carbohydrate antigens below 2 years of age. The carbohydrate antigen only evokes a reaction in the B cells lymphocyte system and T cells (with immunological memory) are not involved. Hence anti capsular opsonic antibodies response, if generated by the antigenic challenge with the vaccine, does not persist beyond 3 months. To be useful in the age group below 2 years, the vaccine would have to be given every 3 months. Hence the only indication of using the A & C vaccine in the age group below 2 years is where an index case is identified in the family. Above the age of 2 years, production of antibody is sustained for at least three years and is useful over a long term, before immunity developes due to subclinical exposure to the organism.

Meningococal vaccine is not recommended to be used below 3 months of age even if there is a family contact. If the epidemic is due to Gr. C meningococcus then it should be remembered that the vaccine is not effective in children below 2 years of age. In fact it may even produce immune tolerance at that age, not allowing successful vaccinations even later. In such cases, chemoprophylaxis is the only answer.

Q.4. What is the efficacy of this vaccine ?

The efficacy of the vaccine is excellent in producing antibodies against group A,C,Y, & W 135. Seroconversion with protective antibody levels develop in over 97% of subjects above 2 years of age.

Unfortunately antibody is not generated against Type B strains, probably due to the neuraminic acid content of the capsular polysaccharide. Adequate antibody levels have been documented upto 7-10 years following vaccination in, U.S.Army recruits.

Q.5. For prevention of epidemic form of meningitis, doctors can take meningococcal vaccine for their own protection. What preventive measure should they take for endemic from of meningitis ?

Endemic meningitis is caused not only by Meningococus but also by pneumococus and Hemo phillus organisms. Precaution need to be taken against all of them.

Ideally doctors should take the pneumococcal polyvalent polysaccharide vaccine along with the Haemophilus influenza b-Protein conjugate vaccine.

However still these diseases are not very contagious and the former 2 vaccines are available with great difficulty in this country. Hence most doctors forego these precautions and do rely on subclinical infections to generate immunity to these diseases.

However a note of caution, with advancing age especially over 65 years the subclinical immunity fades away and resuscitative efforts like suctioning and mouth to mouth breathing for a meningitic patient may impose a heavy bacterial load on the treating health professional. Respiratory precautions and single room isolation for a hospitalised child with pyogenic meningitis, especially in the first 24-48 hours of illness, are very necessary.

If the health professional is inadverantly exposed before a firm diagnosis of pyogenic meningitis is made, he or she would be well advised to take chemoprophylaxis with rifampicin or sulfadiazine.

Q.6. There is a controversy between the use of sulfa and rifampicin for chemoprophylaxis. Kindly clarify. What is the dosage schedule of these drugs ?

Chemoprophylaxis is used to prevent naso-pharngeal carriage of pathogenic microbes in household or close contacts of an index case and thus to prevent secondary cases among the contact. Group A strains of meningococcal meningitis, as were being isolated in Delhi in the recent epidemic, were uniformly susceptible to sulfadiazine. Hence sulfadiazine could widely be used for chemoprophylaxis. However when the organism causing pyogenic meningitis is unknown or is resistant to sulfa (as commonly occurs with type B & C strains) Then rifampicin is a safe alternative in a dose of 20 mg/kg body weight in single daily dose for 2 days. The maximum daily dose of rifampicin should be 600 mg.

Sulfadiazine is used in doses of 1 gm 12 hourly in adults, 500 mg 12 hourly in children between 1 and 12 yrs of age and 500 mg once daily in children below 1 year. Duration of therapy is again 2 days. A brief note here is that trimethoprim sulfa can not be substituted for sulfadiazine since no studies have been done to prove its efficacy. Both sulfadiazine and rifampicin penetrate adequately into oral and naso-pharyngeal secretion and have been shown in field studies to be as effective in eliminating the carrier state.

A number of other antibiotics including the Penicillins which diffuse well in oral secretions and are also used as therapeutic agents in pyogenic meningitis have been shown to be ineffective agents in eliminating nasopharyngeal carriage in field conditions.

Q.7. How can an outbreak of epidemic meningitis be controlled ?

An outbreak of epidemic meningitis can be controlled by the following steps :

i) High index of suspicion in diagnosing meningitis in febrile states.

ii) Respiratory isolation of index patient i.e. a single room with independent air exhaust. All people entering the patients room during first 48 hours must use a disposable mask.

iii) Widespread immunisation in population especially of the household contacts of the index case.

iv) Chemoprophylaxis for household contacts of index case.

Q.8. Can the meningococcal vaccine be used in infants in epidemic situation ?

Group A vaccine is effective for infants from 3 months of age. For children below 18 months, 2 doses at 3 months apart can be given to control the epidemic. Group C component is not effective below 2 years of age.

All children who receive meningococcal vaccine below 2 years of age, should receive a revaccination after 2 years of age to make sure of long term immunity.

Q.9. Meningitis vaccine is not recommended for prevention of endemic form of meningitis. A doctor does not give meningitis vaccination, although it was asked for. Subsequently this child gets meningitis and dies. What is the medico-legal position ?

The medico-legal position is clear. The doctor has given advice based on scentific facts available to him, that the vaccine is not of use in non-epidemic periods.

Subsequently the child dies of meningitis. It is an unfortunate fact, but the doctor cannot be held legally responsible for his advice and suggested course of action.

Q.10. Does a treated case of meningits need vaccination against meningitis ?

Yes. A treated case of meningitis does need vaccination against the disease. Since the occurence of the disease in an individual does not always excite protective antibodies in adequate concentrations. Children have been known to have second and even third episodes of pyogenic meningitis with the same serotype of the organism.

Q.11. What are the contraindications to the use of meningitis vaccination ?

AT : There are no absolute medical contraindications except the presence of fever or a past history of known hypersensitivity to the vaccine. In my opinion a strong contraindication is the inappropriate use of the vaccine on an unsuspecting population without understanding the basis of vaccination used.

ATP : Safety in pregnant women is not established as yet.

Q.12. Can meningitis and typhoid vaccine be given concurrently as recommended after the age of 2 years ?

ATP : Yes, they can be given concurrently since field studies have now shown that the body can respond well to simultaneously administerd antigens.

AT : However I believe no specific study has evaluated the antibody response to an individual antigen after the simultaneous administration of meningococcal and typhoid vaccine.

If there is no compelling need, it is preferable to delay the typhoid vaccine and to give the same after 4 weeks of the meningococal vaccine.

Q.13. What is the dosage schedule in different age groups ?

Uniform dosage schedule of 50 μg of each antigen (A and C) is recommended for all age groups.

Q.14. How often should the meningitis vaccine be repeated ?

Since a single dose itself is immunogenic to the tune of 95% within about 1 week and since the vaccine has been mostly used to control epidemics, the number and intervals of boosters have not been established.

Q.15. In an epidemic situation should we give the vaccine to the whole population or only to the selected high risk groups ?

It is enough if the vaccine is given only to the selected high risk groups.

Q.16. If there is a shortage of vaccine, one would like to give it to only high risk groups. Which are these groups ?

The high risk groups are :

i) Household contacts.

ii) Day care centre contacts.

iii) School contacts.

iv) Medical personnel with intimate exposure.

v) Person in contact with oral secretion of affected patients.

Bibliography

1. M. Pontecorve Report of the committee on Infectious disease. American Academy of Pediatrics 1986 Edition.
2. Pettola H, Kayhty H et al: Meningoccus group A vaccine in children three to five years of age J. Pediatr 1978, 92:818.
3. Roche Scanner Vol. 8 No. 5
4. Vaccines, Sera Immunoglobulin, A practical hand book 1985. Minerva Medical Publishers.
5. Wolfe M.S. Vaccine for foreign travel PCNA 1990, 37:757-769.

NEWER VACCINES 12

Dr. S.K. Mittal & Dr. S. Kukreja

Q.1. What improved vaccines are likely to be available in the coming years ?

Improved versions of several vaccine are likely to become available for general use within this decade. Some of these are :

i) Hepatitis B vaccine : Yeast derived Recombinant DNA vaccine (Engerix-B) against Hepatitis B has largely replaced the plasma derived vaccine available earlier.

ii) Oral typhoid vaccine : Vaccines derived from Ty 21A strain of Salmonella *typhi has* udergone extensive trials and has now received approval by the FDA, USA. Similarly Vi antigen typhoid injectable vaccine has also undergone extensive clinical trials and is likely to become available in none too distant a future.

iii) E-Z measles vaccine : High dose Edmonston-Zagreb strain has been proven to be effective and safe in immunising infants at 3-4 months of age. This should prove to be especially valuable in developing countries where measles tend to occur much earlier than in the developed countries.

iv) Acellular pertussis vaccine : Concern has been expressed about the high rates of side effects with presently available whole cell pertussis vaccine. Acellular pertussis vaccine has been in use in Japan for children above 2 years for last several years and has proven to be as effective with much less side effects. Progress has also been made in developing vaccines from other immunogenic (and not toxigenic) components of pertussis bacilli and these should also be available in near future.

v) Enhanced potency-inactivated polio vaccine (IPV-Ep): This vaccine with the polio content of 40D, 8 D & 32D against type I, II & III respectively has been found to be highly efficacious providing almost 100% protection even with 2 doses given 8 weeks apart. It does not have problem of cold chain storage. This vaccine has already been sanctioned for general use in USA and is scheduled to be manufactured in India also.

All these vaccines are described in details in the respective chapters.

Q.2. Which new vaccines will be received by children and adults in the coming decade ?

Several new vaccines are likely to be available in the near future and may be even included in the routine immunisation schedules. Among these are :

i) Hemophilus influenza B Vaccine
ii) Pneumococcal vaccine
iii) Varicella vaccine
iv) Hepatitis A vaccine
v) Rota virus vaccine
vi) CMV vaccine
vii) Herpes simplex vaccine
viii) HIV-1 vaccine
ix) E. Coli vaccines
x) Leprosy vaccine
xi) Malaria vaccine

Q.3. What are the strategies being used to develop live viral vaccines in future ?

A deeper understanding of the detailed structure of the bacteria and virus and advances in molecular biology has revolutionized development of new vaccines. Several new approaches, incorporating techniques of molecaler engineering have made it possible to develop newer and safer vaccines at a much cheaper rates.

Traditionally live altenuated vaccines have been prepared by passage of live organisms through a series of (relatively) resistant hosts (e.g. BCG) or modification by repeated passage in cell-culture (OPV). Another technique applied was utilisation of variant viruses (e.g. Cow pox virus for small pox vaccine).

All these techniques, although still in use are cumbersome, time consuming and comparatively costly.

The recent molecular techniques being employed for live vaccines are :

a) **DNA modification mutants :** Complete mapping of the viral genomes and the ability to modify directly the structure of the virus at the molecular level has enabled the scientists to develop newer mutant genes of virus which retain immunogenicity while shedding off their virulence. This is done by constructing the DNA genome of the virus in such a way that the key portions which are capable of producing virulence are deleted from the gene. The deletion is done is such a way that reversion of the attenuated form to a virulent form becomes a highly unlikely event. This DNA modification technique is now being used for producing many live virus vaccines for human use.

b) **DNA recombinant vaccine :** The second molecular approach for the development of live attenuated viral vaccine employs the use of non pathogenic virus (vaccinia) as vector (i. e a carrier) for other genes (from viruses against whose protective immune response is to be achieved). The region of vaccinia virus which is non essential for replication is identified and replaced by a part of the gene of another virus against whom immunisation is to be achieved. This part of the gene contains informational elements to produce only the protective antigen of infectious disease pathogen, to excite a protective immunoresponse when administered. The vaccinia virus with this informational gene of foreign virus is grown in cell culture resulting in creation of recombinant virus vaccine.

Vaccines against several viruses like CMV, HIV-I etc. are being developed using this technique and this technique holds great potential in future.

Q.4. What about killed vaccines'. Can advances in moleculor engineering technology be used to produce these vaccines also ?

Yes, moleculor engineering technology has been used to prepare killed vaccines also. Prime example is that of yeast fermented R-DNA vaccine for hepatitis B. Here the surface antigen (HBsAg) gene of hepatitis B is incorporated into a yeast cell (Figure 1). The yeast cell is then fermented ,which allows incorporated surface antigen gene also to be replicated. After fermentation, the surface antigen is separated from yeast debris and purified for use as a vaccine. The advantage of this technique is that one gets large quantity of purified antigen and one does not have to depend on human

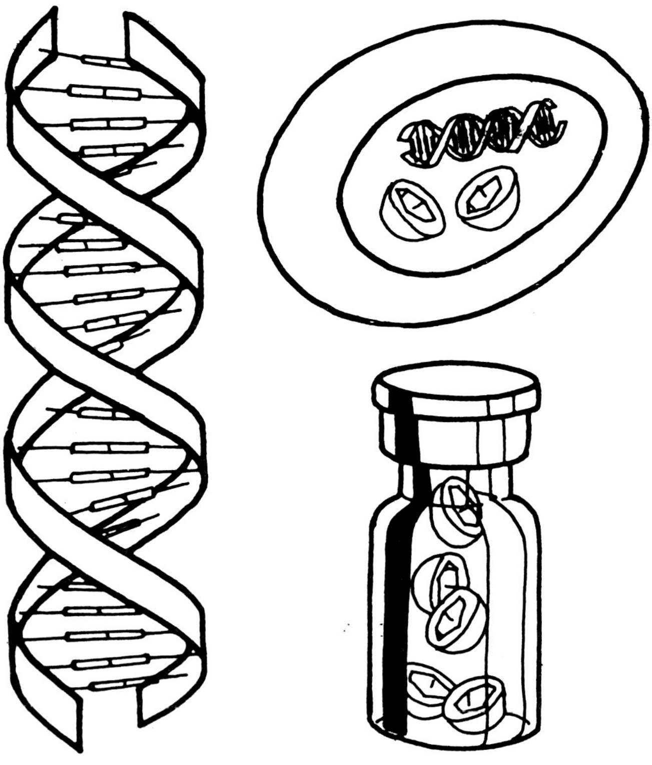

Fig. 1 :– Recombinant-DNA principle in preparing Hepatitis B vaccine

plasma. This molecular approach to vaccine production is known as recombinant derived protein technique. This technique is being used to produce potential vaccines against malaria, leprosy, AIDS, etc. also.

Q.5. Hemophilus influenzae b vaccine has been available in USA since 1985. Yet it did not prove very popular. What are the reasons for this ?

Hemophillus influenzae b vaccine (Hib) utilized the capsular polysaccharide polyribosyl Ribitol Phosphate (PRP) antigen of the organism. This poly-saccharide antigen cannot usually be recognised by infants less than 2 years of age. So this vaccine could be given only at or after 2 years of age. It had a protective efficacy of over 90% but yet it did not help in decreasing the severity or fatality of the disease. It was realised that this was largely due to the fact that most (75%) of the Hib infections occured in children less than 2 years of age and so the vaccine despite being effective, did not become popular.

Q.6. What modifications have been made in the Hib vaccine to over come this shortcoming ?

The polysaccharide antigen of Hib vaccine has been combined with a protein antigen of Diphtheria (PRP-D), Tetanus (PRP-T) or outer membrane Protein of *N. meningitides* (PRP-OMP) to overcome this problem. The infant's immune system is quite capable of recognising these protein antigens and as the polysacecharide antigen is tagged to that protein, it also gets recognised by the host. The polysaccharide antigen (PRP) is a T cell independent antigen but once tagged with protein antigen becomes T-cell dependent antigen. These conjugate vaccine of Hib (PRP-D) has been found to be quit effective and have now been sanctioned for general use in infants in USA and should help greatly in decreasing the high mortality due to this infection.

Q.7. How relevant is Hib vaccine in the context of our country ?

The exact epidemiology of HiB infection in our country is not yet clear. It is largely because it is a fastidious organism to grow. Nevertheless, it is believed to be an important cause of endemic meningitis in our country and more importantly of bacterial pneumonias which are the usual cause of death in acute respiratory infections. Thus Hib vaccine (diphtheria toxoid tagged) has the potential of being in-corporated in the EPI schedule esp. in the context of ARI control programme in our country.

Q.8. What about Pneumococcal vaccine ? How effective is it and what are the indications of its use ?

There are at least 28 serotypes of *strep pneumoniae* capable of causing disease. A vaccine has been produced which incorporates antigen of 14 common pathogenic serotypes of *Pneumococci*. This vaccine is also based on capsular polysaccharide antigen and hence cannot be used in children less than 2 years of age. It is not yet recommended for general use but only in high risk situations. These high risk situations are :

i) Nephrotic Syndrome
ii) Splenectomised children
iii) Sickle cell disease.

Q.9. Chicken pox is such a common disease. Why is there no vaccine against this disease ?

A live attenuated varicella vaccine was developed in Japan in early 1970's. The vaccine is being used in Japan, Korea and other European countries.

Q.10. Why this vaccine is still not in general use ?

The vaccine is still not recommended for general use despite the fact that it is a highly effective vaccine. The reasons for these are :

i) Rather mild nature of chicken pox in children.

ii) Concern regarding duration of immunity

iii) Concern regarding incidence of Zoster after vaccination.

Q.11. What is the present status of this vaccine ?

Recent studies indicate that varicella vaccine is not only high effective (almost 100%) but also the immunity induced once lasts for at least 10 years. Further a follow up of of more than 3300 vaccinated children for 3-4 years showed that only 2 children developed mild zoster during follow up. These two observations have opened up the possibility of this vaccine being used routinely in healthy children. This may be available in combination with MMR as MMRV vaccine.

The greater role of this vaccine at present is its use in immunocompromised individuals, particularly in leukemia. The vaccine has been shown to be quite effective and safe even in immunocompromised individuals and helps to prevent chicken pox which often proves fatal in these individuals.

Bibliography

1. American Academy of Pediatrids, Committee on Infectious Diseases : *Haemophilus influenzae* type b vaccine. Pediatrics 1985, 76:322.
2. American Academy of Pediatrics, Committee on Infectious Diseases: Haemophilus influenzae type b conjugate vaccines: Update. Pediatrics 1989, 84:386.
3. Arbeter AM, Starr SE, Plotkin SA: Varicella vaccine studies in healthy children and adults. Pediatrics 1986, 78:748.
4. Arbeter AM, Baker L, Starr SE, et al: Combination measles, mumps, rubella, and varicella vaccine. Pediatrics 1986, 78:742.
5. Arvin AM, Koropchak CM, Williams BR, et al: Early immune response in healthy and immunocompromised subjects with primary varicella-zoster virus infection. J Infect Dis 1986, 154:422.

6. Asano Y, Itakura N, Hiroishi Y, et al: Viral replication and immunologic responses in children naturally infected with varicella zoster virus and in varicella vaccine recipients. J Infect Dis 1985, 152:863.
7. Asano Y, Nagai T, Miyata T, et al: Long-term protective immunity of recipients of the OKA strain of live varicella vaccine. Pediatrics 1985, 75:667.
8. Bellanti JA. Basic immunological principles. PCNA 1990, 37:513-30.
9. Brunell PA, Novelli VM, Lipton SV, et al: Combined vaccine against measles, mumps, rubella, and varicella, Pediatrics 1988, 81:779.
10. Einhorn MS, Weiberg GA, Anderson E: Immunogenicity in infants of *Haemophilus influenzae* type b polysaccharide in a conjugate vaccine with *Neisseria meningitidis* outer-membrane protein. Lancet 1986, 2:299.
11. Ellis RW: New technologies for making vaccines. In plotkin SA, Mortimer E.A. Jr (eds): Vaccines. Philadelphia, WB Saunders, 1988.
12. Eskola J, Kayhty H. et al: Antibody levels achieved in infants by a course of H. Influenzae type b polysaccharide/diphtheria toxoid conjugate vaccine. Lancet 1985, 1:1184.
13. Eskola J. Peltola H, Takala AK, et al: Efficacy of Haemophilus influenzae type b polysaccharide-diptheria toxoid conjugate vaccine in infancy. N Engl J Med 1987, 317:717.
14. Gelb L, Dohner D, Gershon A, et al: The molecular epidemiology of live attenuated varicella vaccine in children with leukemia and normal adults. J Infect Dis 1987, 155:633.
15. Gershom AA, Viral vaccine of the future. PCNA 1990; 37:689-704.
16. Johnson CE, Shurin PA, Fattlar D, et al: Live attenuated varicella vaccine in healthy 12 to 24 month old children. Pediatrics 1988, 81:512.
17. Lepow ML, Samuelson JS, Gordon LK: Safety and immunogenicity of H, influenza type b polysaccharide-diphtheria toxoid conjugate vaccine in 2 to 6 month old infants. Pediatrics 1987, 80:283.
18. Peltola H, Kayhty H, Sivonen A, et al: Haemophilus influenzae type b capsular polysaccharide vaccine in children: A double-blind field study of 100,000 vaccinees 3 months to 5 years of age in Finland, Pediatrics 1977, 60:730.
19 Shapiro ED: New Vaccine against HiB. PCNA 1990, 37:567-583.

PREVENTION OF DISEASE IN HOUSEHOLD CONTACTS 13

Dr. S.K. Mittal & Dr. S. Kukreja

When one of the child in family in having an infectious disease, very common question which a practitioner has to answer is - What precautions can be taken to prevent this disease in other siblings of the child? A judicious use of public health measures (isolation, excreta disposal etc), immunoglobulins, vaccine and even specific drugs can help to prevent the occurence of disease among household contacts. The steps required for different diseases are different and hence they would be considered separately. It should be remembered however that the disease spreads only to susceptible individuals and if a full course of all vaccines is given to all children at proper ages, the number of suspectible individuals can be substantially decreased.

DIPHTHERIA

1. Patient should be isolated as long as he is infectious (3 consecutive throat swabs negative). Patients must recieve a complete course of penicillin.

2. Fully immunized contacts should receive a booster of D T (<7 yrs of age) or Td (>7 yrs of age), if not given a dose of Diphtheria toxoid within the last 5 years.

3. Unimmunised or partially immunised contacts should have a throat swab culture and be started on chemoprophylaxis at the same time. For chemoprophylaxis, one can give either Inj. Penidure L.A. (0.6 mega units <6 yrs and 1.2 mega units > 6 yrs) or oral erythromycin (30 mg/kg/day×7 days). If the throat swab is positive, then the person can either be a carrier or a new case. This can be distinguished by doing a Schick test which will be positive in a new case and negative in a carrier. This test is however not usually available. Clinically, if the contact with positive throat swab culture is asymptomatic, then he can be continued

treatment as a carrier (erythromycin for 7 days) but if symptoms develop then he should be treated as a case of diphtheria with ADS.

4. Active immunization of the case and all contacts, must be ensured after the attack has been treated.

PERTUSSIS (Whooping cough)

1. For the patient, erythromycin (30-50/kg/dayx7 days) helps to curtail the infectivity of the individual.

2. For contacts<3 months of age, give immediate chemoprophylaxis with erythromycin (30 mg/kg/dayx10 days) and then start active immunization, if child remains asymptomatic.

3. For older infants and children <7 years of age, check immunization status, if completely immunised but have not received a dose of DPT within the last 6 months, then give a dose of DPT together with erythromycin. Otherwise give only erythromycin for 10 days.

4. For children >7 yrs of age, give only erythromycin for 10 days.

TETANUS

Tetanus does not spread to close contacts, so no prophylactic treatment as such is required. Nevertheless occurence of such a case in the family should help to reinforce value of active immunisation against this disease.

MEASLES

For infants <6 months, no specific preventive measures are required. For older contacts: during early contact (<72hrs), measles vaccine (one dose) should be given and the child observed. The child may not develop the disease or develop a mild disease. During late contact (>72hrs), Inj. gammaglobulin may be given but may not be fully effective. It should be followed by active immunisation 12 weeks later. The dose of gamma globulin (16.5%) recommended for preventing an attack of measeles is 0.06 ml/kg. A dose of 0.02 ml/kg of the same, would help to attenuate the disease.

POLIO

All under five children in contacts should be given a dose of OPV irrespective of the immunisation status. Further doses should be given as required to complete the immunisation schedule.

TYPHOID

The patient should be isolated and sanitary disposal of his excreta should be ensured. Contacts should not share food and water with the case. No specific preventive measures are available.

CHOLERA

Isolation of patient and other precautions as for other infections which spread by orofecal route (see Typhoid) should be taken. Tetracycline (Doxicycline 6 mg/kg. O.D.x2 days) is recommended for all household contacts.

INFECTIOUS HEPATITIS

1. All precautions as for other diseases which spread by orofecal route. Patients are infectious till one week after the onset of jaundice.

2. Gammaglobulin to house hold contacts (0.02 ml/kg/stat) has been found to be very effective, but considering that this disease is highly endemic in this country and usually spreads by contaminated (communal) water supply, exposure to this disease is continuous in our country and hence the value of this gammagobulin is routine clinical practice may be suspect.

3. Vaccination against hepatitis A is not available.

4. If the jaundiced person is found to have HBs Ag (Austraila antigen) in blood, then all contacts should receive HBIG,

0.06 ml/kg I.M. stat, together with Hepatitis B vaccine (HBV) at 0, 1 and 6 months (See chapter on Hepatitis). Usually avaiable gammagobulin is not helpful, so if HBIG is not available, give only HBV.

MENINGITIS

Epidemic meningitis is due to Gr. *A or C meningococcus.* Most endemic meningitis are due to *Gr B, meningococcus pneumococcus* or *H.* influenzae infection. No vaccine is available for *GrB meningococcus.* Vaccines against. *H. influenzae b* and *Pneumococcus* are now available in USA and can be imported if required.

Meningococcal Meningitis

For Meningococcal meningitis due to Group A or C meningococcus, chemoprophylaxis with either sulfadiazine (500 mg B.D. x2 days, <6 yrs and 1gm B.D. x 2 days, >6 yrs) or rifampicin (20 mg/kg/day x 2 days, maximum 600 mg/day) to all household contacts should be given. Meningococcal vaccine is recommended for all household contacts (>3 months of age) together with chemoprophylaxis, for preventing epidemic Group A meningococal meningitis. If Group C *meningcoccus* is the infectious agent then the vaccine should be given only to contacts above 2 years of age.

H. Influenzae Meningitis

Chemoprophylaxis with rifampicin (20 mg/kg/day x 4 days) should be given to all household contacts less than 4 years old. Parents should be warned of possibility of secondary infection in the household contacts and should be told to closely observe children for early signs and symptoms of the same.

This should be followed by active immunization of children (2-5 yrs of age) with Hib vaccine (if available). The vaccine (tagged with Diphtheria toxoid) has now been recommended for general use in U.S.A

Pneumococcal Meningitis

No specific recommendations are available for preventing infections among household contacts.
High risk contacts (Nephrotic syndrome, splenectomized, sickle cell disease etc.) should receive active immunization against *Pneumococcus.*

MUMPS

1. Isolation of patients should be ensured till the parotid swellings completely subside (or 10 days after the apperance of parotitis, which ever is later).

2. Non specific immunoglobin and even hyperimmune mumps gloublin are not effective in preventing the disease.

3. Mumps vaccine (alone) or as M.M.R has a doubtful role only if it can be given on the Ist day of contact. This is usually not possible, as a case with mumps is infectious even before the parotid swellings appear.

4. Active immunisation of contacts can begin after 4 weeks of the last fecing case.

RUBELLA

It need not be prevented among children as it causes a very mild illness in them.

Pregnant women especially early in pregnancy (<14 wks of gestation) should avoid exposure to rubella, regardless of history of rubella in childhood or rubella vaccination.

If exposed, then antibody titres should be done on emergency basis to determine the immune status.

1. If pregnant mother has adequate antibody levels, then the pregnancy can be continued as she is immune to rubella.

2. If she is susceptible and gives consent for therapeutic abortion if the need be, repeat rubella antibody test after 2 weeks. If there is evidence of infection, then therapeutic abortion is induced, otherwise the pregnancy can continue.

3. If she is found to be susceptible and if therapeutic abortion is unacceptable to her, passive immunization with immune serum globulin (ISG) 20-30 cc I.M. can be given. The mother should be explained that this may not neccessarily prevent fetal malformation.

CHICKEN POX

1. Patients of chicken pox should be isolated till all scabs have formed. Scabs themselves are not infectious.

2. The contacts need not be protected as it is usually a mild infection and provides life long immunity. However certain individuals, who are at increased risks of developing progressive varicella, need protection against chicken pox. Zoster immune globulin, if available, should be given to such individuals in the dose of 125 units (content of 1 vial) per 10 kg body weights by I.M. route. The high risk groups are :

   a) Immunocompromised hosts (malignancy, children receiving steroids or antimetabolites).

   b) Newborns born to mothers with varicella infection.

PROTECTION OF FOREIGN VISITORS 14

Dr. S.K. Mittal & Dr. S. Kukreja

Q.1. What vaccinations are required to be taken by travellers under international health regulations ?

Previously small pox, cholera and yellow fever were essential before foreign travel. However small pox is no more required as the disease has been completely eradicated from the World. Cholera vaccine has gone into disrepute because of its poor efficacy (about 35%) and in 1988, WHO eliminated the requirement of cholera vaccine for international travellers. A few countries still demand cholera vaccination although without much scientific validity.

Yellow fever is the only vaccine required for international travel and that too if one is travelling to and fro its endemic areas.

Q.2. Yellow fever vaccine is required for travel to which countries ?

Yellow fever is endemic mostly in African and South American countries. Only travelles to and from these countries are required to have yellow fever vaccine.

Q.3. Can you tell us something about yellow fever vaccine ?

All children more than 9 months of age travelling to an endemic area should receive yellow fever vaccine in the dose of 0.5 ml subcutaneously. Young children less than 6 months of age should not be given this vaccine as they are at an increased risk of developing encephalits. Simultaneous administration of chloroquine (for malaria prophylaxis) or gammaglobulin (for prophylaxis against hepatitis) does not interfere with the protection offered by yellow fever vaccine. The vaccine provide immunity for 10 years and hence for international certificate of vaccination to remain valid, one requires revaccination every 10 years.

Q.4. One of my friends, a resident in America, is planning to visit India. What advise should I give him so that his family is protected from various infectious diseases ?

Before starting from America (or from any developed country) they must receive:

1. Typhoid vaccination, two doses at 2 weeks interval or oral typhoid vaccine.
2. a dose of gamaglobulin (0.02 ml/kg) for protection against infectious hepatitis. To be repeated if the stay is more than 3 months.
3. Chemoprophylaxis against malaria (weekly choroquin 5 mg/kg) should be started a week prior to their arrival and should be continued till three weeks after return to America.

Q.5. What about the children ? Do the same instructions apply for them also.

It will depend on the age of children :

a) **Upto 1 year of age :** They should get all their routine immunization as per the schedule in their own country which can then be continued in India. A dose of measles vaccine at least 6-8 weeks prior to travel to endemic areas should also be given to infants 6-12 months of age. Immunoglobulin should be given at least 6 weeks after the measles vaccine.

1-5 year : These children would have already received routine immunisation course including MMR in their country. They should be given a dose of Hib vaccine if already not received. They should also receive typhoid vaccination, gammaglobulin and chloroquine prophylaxis.

Older children : As for adults, as described in Q. No. 4.

Q.6. What about BCG vaccine ? Should these children not get BCG vaccination ?

Use of BCG as preventive measure remains controversial. It is generally not recommended. Instead it is recommended to do Mantoux testing (after 12 weeks of return to their country) and then to take appropriate action accordingly.

Q.7. Should these children receive meningococal and JE vaccine also ?

Meningococeal vaccine should be given only if an epidemic situation is prevailing in the area of visit. It is effective within 10 days of administration. (See chapter on Meningococeal vaccine).

Japanese B encephalits vaccine needs to be given if only the area of visit includes countries of South and south East Asia including India particularly if protection from mosquito bites cannot be ensured. In India particularly the States of Andhra, Karnataka and Bihar have a high incidence of this disease, particularly in the breeding season of the mosquitos. The vaccine used is formalin activated mouse brain vaccine made in Japan. 2 doses of vaccine 1 ml. each (0.5 ml for children less than 3 years) administered subcutaneously, at an interval of 7-14 days are required for primary vaccination.

Q.8. Rabies is an endemic disease in many countries including India. Should visitors be protected against this disease ?

Pre-exposure prophylaxis with HDCV is recommended prior to visit to endemic areas only for young children who seem to be at a particularly high risk of contracting the disease because of their fondness of dogs. Pre-exposure prophylaxis does not obviate the need of post-exposure therapy but definitely avoids the need of Human Rabies Immunoglobulin (H.R.I.G.). (For details see chapter on Rabies vaccine).

It must be remembered that simultaneous chloroquine prolohylaxis may interfere with the efficacy of pre exposure rabies prophylylaxis.

Manual UIP, Ministry of Health.

Vaccines must stay cold all the way from the manufacturer to the child. The equipment and the people that keep vaccines cold from the manufacturer to the child are together called THE COLD CHAIN.

1. Before vaccines reach the Health Centre:

* They must be collected quickly from the airport;

* They must be stored at the correct cold temperature in the refrigerator at the Central Store, the Regional Store, and the District Store.

* They must be kept cold during transport form one store to another.

Then vaccines arrive at your Health Centre in good condition.

2. After vaccines reach the Health Centre:

* You must keep them at +4° to +8°C in your Health Centre refrigerator.

* You must carry them to the immunization session in a vaccine carrier with ice or frozen ice packs.

* You must keep the vaccine vials in a cup of ice or on top of an ice pack while you immunise the children.

Looking after vaccines in a Health Centre refrigerator

You can keep vaccines in good condition in a Health Centre refrigerator. But you must look after them carefully. Do not keep more then one months' requirement at any given time.

What damages vaccines

You can easily damage vaccines if you do not look after them carefully.

A vaccine is POTENT, if it is in good condition, and able to make a child immune. If it is damage, and unable to make a child immune, then it has LOST ITS POTENCY.

All vaccines lose their potency after a certain time, even with good care. You know when that time is, from the EXPIRY DATE printed on the vaccine vial.

Heat, sunlight and freezing can all damage vaccines

* Heat and sunlight damage vaccines.

* Freezing damages the killed vaccines and toxoids, like DPT DT, TT and typhoid.

Keep all vaccines at the correct cold temperature, and out of the sunlight.

If a vaccine is damaged by heat or by freezing you cannot make it potent again. It does not help to put it back at the correct temperature after the damage is done.

Arrange the vaccines correctly in the refrigerator

* Stock the vaccines neatly so that air can move between the boxes.

* Keep measles and polio vaccines on the TOP shelf near the freezer.

* Keep DPT, TT, DT and Typhoid on the MIDDLE shelf, so that they are away form the evaporator.

* Keep the diluent (for measles and BCG) in the refrigerator with the vaccine (but not in the freezer).

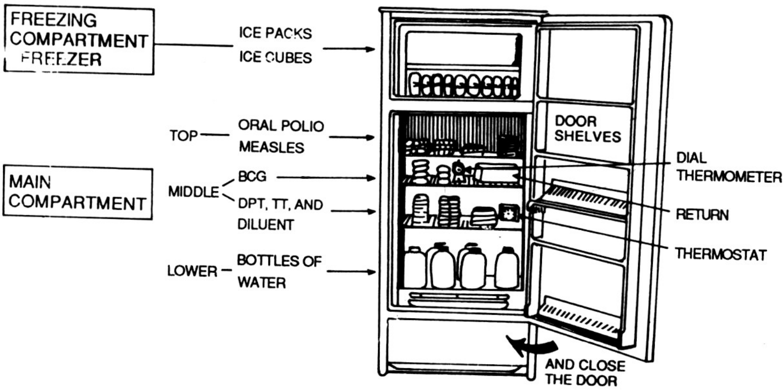

Fig. 1 A Health Centre refrigerator showing vaccine stored correctly.

* Have a special box to keep 'RETURNED' vaccine that has been taken to an immunization session in a vaccine carrier.
* Keep plastic bottles of water or spare ice packs on the LOWER shelf to help to keep the refrigerator maintain low temperature in case of power failure.
* Keep the door close. When you need to open it, plan what you will do first. Then open the door. do what you have to and close the door quickly.

Defrosting the refrigerator

Press the defrost switch. If the refrigerator does not have a defrost switch, unplug the refrigerator.

Wait for 1-2 hours

The ice will automatically melt

The water is collected in the chill tray which is just below the freezer

Remove this tray and throw away the water

Clean the refrigerator with a soft cloth

In refrigerators which have an automatic defrost switch, the refrigerator will automatically start again. If the refrigerator does not have a defrost switch, and you have switched off the electricity, you can now switch it on again.

Put the dial thermometer on the racks, close the door and let the refrigerator run for some time.
Check the temperature on the dial thermometer. If it is +4° to 8°C, transfer the vaccine to the refrigerator.

To defrost the refrigerator faster, you can keep a pot of hot water in the freezer or you can wipe its inner walls with a cloth dipped in hot water.

Never scrape ice form the freezer. Sharp and pointed objects can damage the walls and render the refrigerator useless.

Arrange the vaccine correctly

Check the temperature twice a day

Defrost, if ice more than 1/2 cm thick

Do not keep vaccine stock more than one month

3. Cold chain equipment to transport vaccines

You must keep vaccines cold all the way from the refrigerator to the child or mother, whom you immunize. Vaccine carriers are used for carrying small quantities of vaccines of the sub-centres or villages or to clinics.

Vaccine carriers

Vaccine carriers have thick walls and lids. They are made of special material which does not allow heat to pass through it. Insulation cannot make vaccines cold. Only a refrigerator or ice can make things cold. But an insulated container can keep ice and vaccines cold for a short time, because heat cannot go inside to warm them.

Do not leave vaccine carriers in sunlight

Do not leave the lid open

Do not drop or sit on them

Keep clean and dry

Use frozen ice packs

Ice packs

Cold packs (ice packs) are used for lining the walls of the vaccines carries to keep them cold. They are flat plastic bottles filled with water. The ice packs are prepared by keeping them in the freezer or in the freezer compartment of an ordinary refrigerator. The ice packs should stand with their edges and not flat on one another. This will reduce the time taken to freeze the ice pack. Salt should not be added to the water.

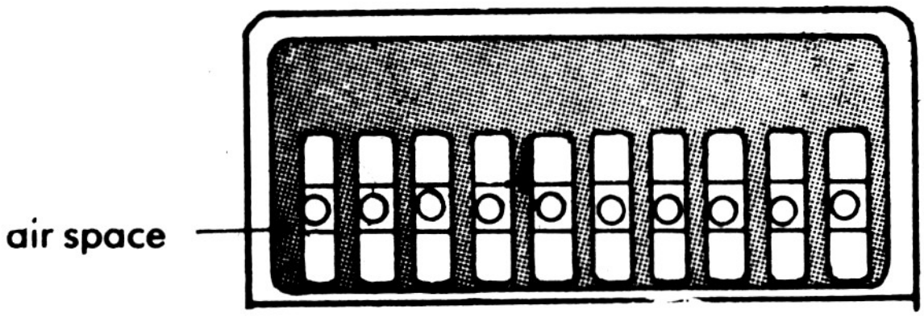

How to prepare ice packs

* Fill the ice pack upto 3 cms from the top with water and put the cap on tightly (see diagram)
* Hold it upside down and shake it to make sure that it does not leak. If it leaks, tighten the cap and shake again to see that it does not leak.
* Put the ice pack or bottle on its side in the freezer.
* Leave the ice pack overnight to freeze solid. Do not put more than 6 packs for freezing at the same time.

Preparing to pack your vaccine carrier

Before you open the refrigerator door :

* Decide how many vials of each vaccine to pack. For this,
  - You need to know how many children you expect to come to the session.
  - You need to know how many doses of vaccine each vial contains
  - You always need a spare vial of vaccine.
  - Take one ampoule of diluent for each vial of measles and BCG.

* Leave vaccines and diluents in the refrigerator until the vaccine carrier is ready.
* Check the vaccine carrier.
  – Check the insulation (for cracks).
  – Check that the lid fits tightly, and that the catches work.

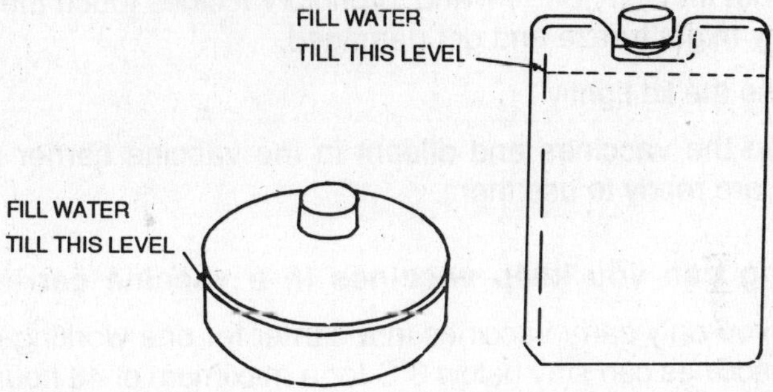

Arranging ice cubes in thermocole box/thermos flask

You must only use ice cubes in plastic bags.

* Put a bag of cubes in the bottom of the carrier
* Put the vaccines on the ice.
* Put a bag of cubes on top of the vaccine

Packing the vaccines

Taking the vaccines out of the refrigerator

* First take the vaccines that you took to your last immunization session but which you did not use. (Keep a special box in the refrigerator marked "RETURN"). Take only as many returned vials out of the refrigerator as you can use during the session.
* Then take the OLDEST vaccines that have been in you refrigerator for the longest time.
* Look at the label of each vial of vaccine and check the expiry date.

If vaccine has passed the expiry date: Do not use it. Take it out of the refrigerator. Record it as "wasted"

* Close the refrigerator door.

Use the return vaccines before the others

Use the oldest vaccines first

Putting the vaccines into the carrier

* Check that the ice packs are full and frozen solid.
* Put newspaper or cardboard or plastic foam all around the DPT, DT, TT and Typhoid vaccines, between them and the ice packs.

  Do not let DPT, DT, TT and Typhoid vaccines touch the ice. They might freeze and get damaged.
* Close the lid tightly
* Keep the vaccines and diluent in the vaccine carrier until you are ready to use them.

How long can you keep vaccines in a vaccine carrier ?

Usually, you only carry vaccines in a carrier for one working day. But the vaccines can stay below 8°C for a maximum of 48 hours if:

- You keep the lid on tightly.
- and you leave all the ice packs and ice cubes inside.

So if you are very careful you can keep vaccines in the carrier for one night and use them the next day.

The vaccines can be kept safely in the vaccine carrier so long as the ice packs have not fully malted.

4. How to keep the vaccine cold on the immunisation table

You must keep opened vaccine vials in a cup or pot of ice, or on ice pack while you immunise.

The ice cubes or an ice pack for the table can come from your vaccine carrier or refrigerator.

Because you take out some of the ice, the inside of the vaccine carrier becomes warm more quickly.

However, the vaccines can stay below 38°C for one working day.